Advance Prais
Tibetan Yo

"Alejandro Chaoul offers the gift of his lifelong passion ancient tradition of Tibetan yoga so that we may all benefit from these practices. Whether you are looking to heal your heart, body, or mind, this book sets forth a clear path to aid in your journey toward wholeness."
—Sharon Salzberg, author of *Lovingkindness* and *Real Change*

"An extraordinary teaching of the inner and secret practices of the Bön tradition's yoga and the power of these practices to awaken and heal."
—Roshi Joan Halifax, abbot, Upaya Zen Center

"I cannot recommend this book highly enough as an authentic, creative, delightful, and powerfully transformative teaching that, if studied and applied sincerely, can change people's lives for the better!"
—Robert Thurman, Buddhologist, author, environmentalist

"Reading *Tibetan Yoga* is equivalent to receiving the transmission of this ancient art directly from the mouth of a master. Chaoul reveals the secret of freedom through motion: how we too can discover magic and wisdom in a way that is accessible, joyful, and liberating."
—Willa Blythe Baker, author of *The Wakeful Body*

"Lucid and accessible, this treasure provides a rare portal to the hidden oral teachings of Tibetan yoga. A remarkable achievement!"
—Acharya Judith Simmer-Brown, PhD, Naropa University, and author of *Dakini's Warm Breath*

"It's wonderful when thirty years of study and practice flow into words that bring an ancient and magnificent tradition to life. These practices combine unique sounds, imagery, and movement as pathways toward a more natural and fundamental sense of being. Clear and authentic."
—Anne C. Klein (Rigzin Drolma), professor, department of religion, Rice University, and founding teacher, Dawn Mountain

"Thorough and accessible, this precious book is a gift that opens us up to the unfamiliar yet profound, ancient teachings of Tibetan yoga. Clear instructions along with commentaries by Tibetan wisdom masters illuminate how these magical movements can clear away obstacles and lead to internal transformation at the deepest level."
—Susan Bauer-Wu, president of the Mind & Life Institute, and author of *Leaves Falling Gently*

"In *Tibetan Yoga*, Alejandro Chaoul masterfully reveals important, yet lesser known, mind-body practices. Chaoul takes us on a beautiful journey that is personal, historical, and practical. *Tibetan Yoga* teaches us how to incorporate these ancient practices into everyday life, resulting in profound improvements in the physical, psychological, and spiritual aspects of our lives."
—Lorenzo Cohen, PhD, professor and director, integrative medicine program, MD Anderson Cancer Center

"*Tibetan Yoga* reveals a treasure trove of simple, deep body practices, which profoundly expand the tools for most contemporary practitioners of meditation. Chaoul is the perfect guide on the journey of embodying this ancient wisdom—his devotion to scholarly and spiritual depth is complemented by his contemporary scientific grounding and expertise as a teacher. This book awakens not only the subtle body but also our sense of wonder and joy as we learn how to become the kestrel, the donkey, the tigress, the peacock, and more!"
—Eve Ekman, PhD, co-creator of the Atlas of Emotions

"A wonderfully illuminating book with exceptionally clear instructions, abundant and interwoven contextualization. Alejandro Chaoul offers a splendid gateway into understanding the 'magical movements' tradition in its theory and practice."
—David Germano, professor of Tibetan Buddhism

TIBETAN YOGA

Magical Movements of Body, Breath, and Mind

ALEJANDRO CHAOUL

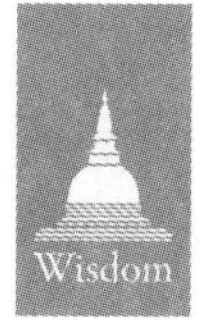

Wisdom Publications
199 Elm Street
Somerville, MA 02144 USA
wisdomexperience.org

Library of Congress Cataloging-in-Publication Data
Names: Chaoul, Alejandro, author.
Title: Tibetan yoga: magical movements of body, breath, and mind / Alejandro Chaoul.
Description: Somerville, MA: Wisdom Publications, [2021] |
Includes bibliographical references.
Identifiers: LCCN 2021024502 (print) | LCCN 2021024503 (ebook) |
ISBN 9781614295228 (paperback) | ISBN 9781614295464 (ebook)
Subjects: LCSH: Qi gong.
Classification: LCC RA781.8 .C434 2021 (print) | LCC RA781.8 (ebook) |
DDC 613.7/1489—dc23
LC record available at https://lccn.loc.gov/2021024502
LC ebook record available at https://lccn.loc.gov/2021024503

ISBN 978-1-61429-522-8 ebook ISBN 978-1-61429-546-4

25 24 23 22 21 5 4 3 2 1

Cover design by Phil Pascuzzo. Interior design by Gopa & Ted 2, Inc.

Line drawings by Isabelle Augé © Adagp 2021. Author photo by Andreas Zihler. Photo of Yongdzin Tenzin Namdak by Rosa María Méndez. Thangka of channels and of Shardza Tashi Gyaltsen by Lharila Kalsang Nyima. Graphic of chakras by Sydney Leijenhorst. Cover image: figure from the Zhang Zhung Aural Transmission Tsakli set, courtesy of Triten Norbutse monastery in Nepal.

Printed on acid-free paper that meets the guidelines for permanence and durability of the Production Guidelines for Book Longevity of the Council on Library Resources.

Printed in the United States of America.

Please visit fscus.org.

I dedicate this book to my teacher Yongdzin Tenzin Namdak Rinpoche.

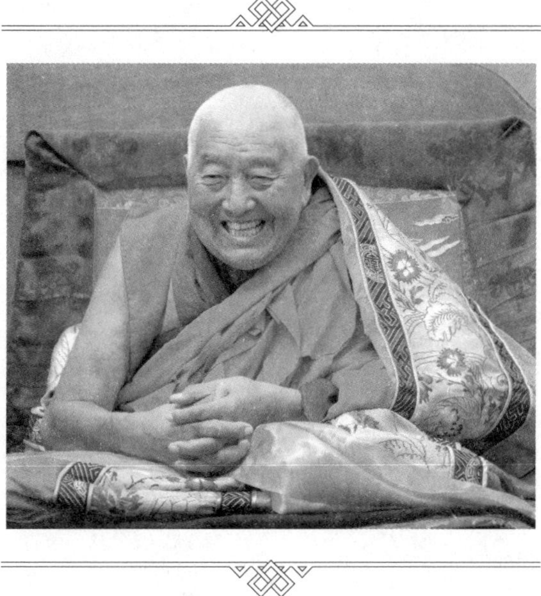

Through him I entered the Bön teachings in 1991, and since then he has been a constant support in my spiritual path.

When I am in difficulties, I hear his words telling me, "Don't forget we are in samsara," and as I visualize him with his wonderful smile, those difficulties and obstacles seem to dissolve like a snowflake in the ocean.

And when that is not enough, I practice these magical movements.

Table of Contents

Foreword

ALEJANDRO (ALE) CHAOUL has been my student for almost thirty years. Not only have I come to know him well as a friend, but I also admire his enduring engagement in Bön study and practice, both personally and academically. From the start Ale has played an important role in the activities of Ligmincha International, including organizing some of our retreats, creating support materials for practice and study, teaching, directing research initiatives and conferences, and otherwise offering his dedicated assistance. He is a graduate of Ligmincha International's seven-year study program, was in the first group of The 3 Doors trainees, and now serves as a senior teacher for Ligmincha International and The 3 Doors.

Ale's passion for the Tibetan yogas of Tsalung Trulkhor was sparked during a visit to Triten Norbutse Monastery in Nepal, where he studied under the supervision of my beloved teacher Yongdzin Tenzin Namdak and Khenpo Nyima Wangyal. After his return to the United States in 1994, I worked closely with him in going over the *Zhang zhung Nyengyu Trulkhor* texts and practices, including Shardza Rinpoche's commentary, to support him in teaching Tibetan yoga and eventually creating a training program for students in the United States, Latin America, and Europe. I share Ale's deep interest in the healing potential of these yogas and I was very happy to support him in bringing these ancient practices into hospitals and other healthcare environments in the form of research studies and clinical applications, as well as in creating conferences and forums of dialogue between scientific and spiritual leaders.

Over the past three decades Alejandro Chaoul has gained an intimate knowledge of Tibetan yoga through his consistent practice: training under many Bön lamas at Triten Norbutse and at Menri Monastery, India, and making Tibetan yoga the topic of his PhD dissertation. His book *Tibetan*

Yoga: Magical Movements of Body, Breath and Mind is the fruit of this knowledge. It offers an accessible and thorough presentation of the *Zhang zhung Nyengyu Trulkhor*, or *Tibetan Yoga of the Zhang Zhung Aural Transmission*. I am sure it will shed a lot of light on Tibetan yoga for those interested in the topic and will do much to deepen the experiences of those practicing it.

Geshe Tenzin Wangyal Rinpoche

Preface: A City Yogi

I WAS BORN in Argentina, a very Catholic country, into a Jewish family that sent me to a Presbyterian school so I would learn English. These were great opportunities to absorb different spiritual traditions, but none resonated with me for very long. It was college that opened my eyes, my mind, and my heart. I took courses in Indian philosophy, Asian religions, and became friends with students of many countries, being drawn particularly to those from India. Outside of school, there were opportunities for free classes, and I took advantage of them. I learned photography, yoga, Zen meditation, and vegetarian cooking with the Hare Krishna. When I graduated, I got my backpack and headed to India. In my nine months of gestation there, many things flourished, and many waned. I initially went to meet some of my college friends, but more importantly I went to meet myself.

Circumstances and traumas in my life had pulled me to India and Nepal, drawing me in search of the mirror of my soul. My Indian friends told me I would come across many charlatans that pass as teachers and warned me to be cautious as I journeyed throughout the country in my spiritual quest. I was fascinated by wonderful people from all different traditions: Hindus, Sikhs, Jains, Buddhists, Muslims, as well as Christians and Jews. And I did meet many teachers, learning from all of them, whether or not I stayed on with them.

My encounter with U.G. Krishnamurti shattered all my philosophical beliefs that my years as an undergrad had led me to construct. Letting them go was a welcome relief. However, asking what to do next, U.G.'s simple response of "just be" was too profound for me to understand. Since I didn't know how to be, even though it seemed an important thing to accomplish, I thanked him and continued my journey. I went to an ashram that some of my Hindu friends endorsed and met the main teacher, Swami Chinmayananda, a wonderful and cheerful human being, full of knowledge and compassion. I became interested in his teachings and his program, and I was particularly captivated by his own story: as a young Indian independence activist and journalist he had set out to expose the Himalayan swamis, the holy men who attracted crowds of disciples but who, the young skeptic thought, were greedy charlatans. He went to interview Swami Sivananda at his ashram in Rishikesh and was utterly transformed. Leaving off his worldly inquiry, he turned his attention toward his own mind and went on to become one of India's greatest Vedanta teachers. He was the first teacher to exemplify for me the importance of skepticism and exploring the nature of one's own existence.

I also met Tibetan Buddhists as I walked in the mountainous region of Ladakh, visiting many monasteries where the monks offered me food and a place to stay, showing me their butter-lamp-lit altars with many figures and always a photo of His Holiness the Dalai Lama—of whom I then knew very little. After a Hindu pilgrimage to Amarnath Cave, and a period of time with Sikhs at the Golden Temple in Amritsar, I was hosted by a Muslim family in the saffron-growing region of Kashmir. While bicycling from Pampore to Srinagar I saw, on the front page of an Indian newspaper in English, the announcement that the Dalai Lama had been awarded the Nobel Peace Prize. I felt happy, as if my own mom or dad had been the awardee. As I stayed in the region, I grew to be even more attracted toward the Tibetan people and their spiritual leader and decided to pursue that interest. And I felt supported by Swami Chinmayananda in this choice. When I told him I wanted to follow the Dalai Lama, he fed me *prasad* (blessed food) and gracefully said, "There is no coming or going, all is *maya*, an illusion; go on, my son." I left with this blessing, and this blessed journey still goes on, my small part in the endless unfolding of *maya.*

Thus I made my way to Dharamsala, where I arrived in time to join the celebrations of the fortieth anniversary of the Tibetan Children's Village School, one of the first and strongest institutions of the Tibetan exile community. There, I was not only stunned by His Holiness's presence—in my excitement I was shaking, so none of my photos came out—but also the children who gave me a great lesson when, at the end of their performance, they stood in the courtyard together, all dressed in white, and then curled their bodies to form the phrase "Others before Self."

This resonated with the wonderful hospitality I received in the monasteries and in the houses where I stayed, in the Tibetan restaurants and tea shops—really everywhere. I started having that warm feeling of being home, and in an odd way it came to feel even more familiar than my home back in Buenos Aires.

I was so touched by these people who opened their homes, monasteries, and shops with a warm smile that came from deep in their heart—it was an inexplicable sense of being welcomed. I was also able to see His Holiness in a public blessing, after which I was speechless and silently absorbing the experience as tears of inexplicable joy ran down my cheeks. Before I left, I heard him say, "A good heart is the best religion." It is a phrase that keeps ringing true in me, and it has been an anchor in tempestuous times.

My relationship with Tibetan lamas continued to deepen. I found my first teacher, Yeshe Dorje Rinpoche, in Zilnon Kagye Ling Monastery in Dharamsala. I then studied with Namkahi Norbu Rinpoche at the Tashigar Center in Argentina. Rinpoche directed me to Lopon Tenzin Namdak, who gave one of the lectures before His Holiness the Dalai Lama presided over the Kalachakra initiation in Madison Square Garden in New York City, in October 1991.

Each of these teachers struck "home" in their own unique ways to help me in my spiritual journey. I received the preliminary practices of the Nyingma tradition from Yeshe Dorje Rinpoche and I committed to finishing its 100,000 repetitions—and actually, following his advice, did 111,111 repetitions of each practice. In the seven years that I took to complete it, I continued to take teachings with my lamas, and became even more deeply acquainted with Dzogchen and the Bön tradition.

Someone in India had told me, referring to the exploration of different traditions, that it was good to dig in many holes, but that once you get to the water, keep digging in that one. So it was for me in the Bön tradition.

After the 1991 Kalachakra, smitten with Lopon Tenzin Namdak, I went to visit him at his monastery in Nepal, Triten Norbutse. In 1993 I was in the

US again, and I heard that Tenzin Wangyal Rinpoche was teaching in New Mexico. I met him during Losar, the Tibetan New Year; meeting Tenzin Wangyal Rinpoche began not just a new year, but truly a new life!

That summer I went to the University of Virginia for a summer intensive Tibetan language class and found that Tenzin Wangyal Rinpoche was in Charlottesville. We met again and he invited me to the seven-year study program he was starting, in which, I was overjoyed to hear, Lopon Tenzin Namdak would be playing a major role.

When I saw these two lamas teaching together, so beautifully embodying the teacher–student relationship, it was as though all the Bön masters from the past had come alive. I had such a vivid feeling in my whole body, tingling and almost sweating, feeling the hairs in my arms rising as though electrified. My breath was full and my mind clear. At that moment I realized that I had found the water; this was the lineage in which to dig deep.

Rinpoche and Lopon were both very supportive of my desire to pursue my academic studies focusing in Tibetan religions. So, after an MA at the University of Virginia, I did a PhD at Rice University, with a dissertation on the magical movements teaching of the *Zhang Zhung Aural Transmission*. During that time both my father and Namkhai Norbu Rinpoche were diagnosed with cancer, and I was inspired to begin volunteering at the MD Anderson Cancer Center, teaching meditation to people with cancer and to their caregivers, which I did under the supervision of Tenzin Wangyal Rinpoche. A year later, together with Lorenzo Cohen, a researcher at MD Anderson, we formed a team researching the possible benefits of Tibetan Yoga for people with cancer. When Lorenzo, Rinpoche, and I met, it felt like a dream team. Lorenzo asked Rinpoche what would be the most important aspect to measure, and without hesitation Rinpoche said "openheartedness." Although this isn't something that has a clear metric—as Lorenzo mentioned—Rinpoche's answer struck a chord in us and offered further confirmation that we were continuing to dig in the right direction. As His Holiness had said almost a decade earlier, "A good heart is the best religion," and so openheartedness seemed the right way to go

It was from His Holiness the Dalai Lama, in the 1990 Losar teachings at Namgyal Monastery in Dharamsala, that I had first heard teachings on the *Six Yogas of Naropa*. This was my first introduction to a Tibetan style of yoga. The *six yogas* does not refer to "yoga" in the way we think of it in the West, but it does include some of the magical movements—*trulkhor*—that would become the focus of my studies and which are the subject of this book. Tibetan yoga, like the classical Indian traditions, is a whole-being practice, involving both mind and body. His Holiness the Dalai Lama further encouraged me during his first visit to South America, when he told me that Tibetan medicine was a wonderful way to introduce Dharma in a peaceful and holistic way. That planted a seed. With the work in the hospitals, I was able to include a section in my dissertation on the applications of Tibetan yoga in contemporary medicine, particularly focusing on people with cancer and how it affects their quality of life. Our first research study was published in 2004 and I completed my dissertation in 2006. We continued with the research.

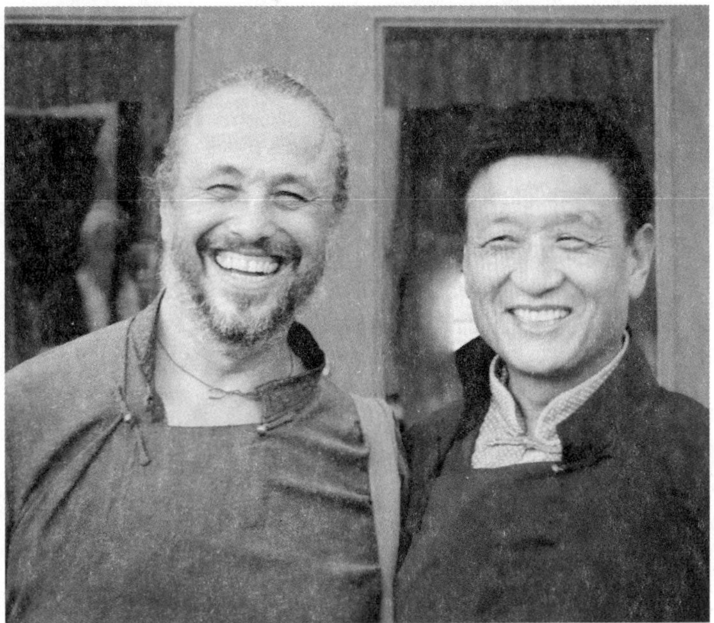

Tenzin Wangyal Rinpoche and Alejandro Chaoul at Ligmincha International's Twenty-Fifth Anniversary

This book is the result of the work on my dissertation and the subsequent research as well as the years of learning and teaching these practices within

Ligmincha International—the community established by Tenzin Wangyal Rinpoche—as well as yoga and meditation centers and healthcare facilities. I am grateful to my teachers, family, students, patients, and caregivers for all that they have taught me, which I humbly pass on to others with this book.

NOTE: While this book introduces the practice and provides a framework for the concepts of magical movement, a direct oral explanation from a teacher is still necessary to master them.

Acknowledgments

I AM GRATEFUL to this wonderful lineage that was transmitted from the mouth of a teacher, through a bamboo cane, to the ear of the disciple (i.e., aurally transmitted—*nyen gyu*), and then, luckily for us, expanded as they were written down, and still transmitted, in this aural, magical way.

To all the masters of these Zhang Zhung Aural Transmission magical movements, starting with Pongyal Tsenpo down to Yangton Chenpo and Bumje Ö, and centuries later to Shardza Tashi Gyaltsen.

And particularly, the contemporary masters like Yongdzin Tenzin Namdak—for escaping Tibet, helping these teachings survive, and passing them on to those he trained in exile in India and Nepal. Under his supervision and that of Nyima Wangyal, then the *khenpo* of Triten Norbutse Monastery, I learned these magical movements with a young monk recently arrived from Tibet, Y Tenzin. I am incredibly grateful to them, as they planted the seed that became a central part of my life, both as a heart practice and an academic pursuit.

To Tenzin Wangyal Rinpoche, I cannot find enough words to say THANK YOU! My continuous mentor, both spiritually and academically, who, when I returned to see him after I learned these practices, met with me every day at 5 a.m. to go over them and Shardza's *Commentary*. He encouraged me to deepen my study and practice not just with him but also with his teachers in the United States and in their monasteries in India and Nepal, making sure that I learned thoroughly and guiding me so I can teach others.

To Menri Ponlob Trinley Nyima, for his teachings and numerous discussions both in Menri Monastery in India, as well as in Ligmincha International in Virginia, and in Houston. And to Khenpo Tenpa Yungdrung, for his teachings and discussions in Triten Nobutse, in Shenten Dargye Ling in

France and in Ligmincha International. As well as many other teachers of this tradition that helped me learn and deepen these magical movements: Geshe Yungdrung Gyaltsen, Geshe Tenzin Yangton, and Geshe Tenzin Yeshe, among others.

And of course, too, to the late His Holiness Lungtok Tenpa Nyima, the Thirty-Third Menri Trizin, for his teachings and support, particularly during my magical movement retreat based on Shardza's *Main Points* at Menri Monastery.

To all of them, I thank them from my heart, through my daily prostrations, as I take refuge, and my magical movement practice.

To the Western scholars that helped me shape what I had learned, studied, and practiced into my PhD dissertation in 2006: Anne Klein, David Germano, Edith Wyschogrod, William Parsons, Richard Smith, Jeffrey Kripal, and Andrew Fort.

And now, as it takes shape as this book, fifteen years later, my immense gratitude to the Wisdom Publications team, starting with Daniel Aitken, who surprised me when he showed interest in my work and even read my dissertation, and then brought his team to make it into this book; to Laura Cunningham, who became the editorial manager; and Rory Lindsay, the general editor, with whom I had countless emails that helped shape this book. To Emma Varvaloucas, who helped me with the introduction and Alexander Gardner, whom I knew from our grad-student days, and who became an incredible help editing this book into what you are reading today. Kestrel Montague and Patty McKenna have been wonderful in coordinating the marketing and Kestrel was also superb in bringing ideas back and forth to Phil Pascuzzo, who designed an amazing cover, extending to the back. And to Ben Gleason, who coordinated the interior design and proofreading. A truly amazing team that I am sure also include others that I don't get to interact with, and so I thank you all for helping this book manifest.

This book would also not be what it is without the help of a long-time friend, Kurt Keutzer, who came into this project in its last two months, and in that crunch helped me to comprehensively edit the translation of Shardza's *Commentary* that you see in appendix 1. I don't have enough words to thank him for so many hours and days, my back-and-forth questions, and the impact that the changes we made in the translation had on the rest of the book. My thanks to Kurt also for his generosity in allowing me to include in appendix 2 the translation of Shardza's *Tsalung Söldep* (Channels-and-Winds Prayer) that he and Geshe Chaphur Lhundup did. Thank you both.

Special thanks to everyone who allowed me to use the photos and graphics: Rosa Maria Méndez, for the beautiful photo of Yongdzin Tenzin Namdak for the dedication of this book; to Lharila Kalsang Nyima for the painting of the channels as well as the thangka of Shardza Rinpoche he painted for Raven Cypress Wood, and to Raven for sending me the wonderful photo of it; to Sydney Leijenhorst for the graphic of the chakras; to Isabelle Augé for the line drawings of meditation postures; to Samten Karmay for all his support and giving me permission to use the image of Togme Zhigpo from his *Little Luminous Boy*; to Triten Norbutse for all the *tsakli* images of Aural Transmission masters; and to Eddy Philippe for his skillful help in the digital editing all of these images.

And to friends, teachers, and colleagues whom I admire. Thank for your kind endorsements for this book: Roshi Joan Halifax, Sharon Salzberg, Bob Thurman, Willa Blythe Miller, Judith Simmer-Brown, Eve Ekman, Lorenzo Cohen, Susan Bauer-Wu, David Germano, Cyndi Lee, and Anne Klein, as well as Mary Taylor and Richard Freeman. And to my students and friends Rob Patzig and Gigi Falk for reading different parts of the manuscript and providing valuable suggestions. A deep bow and gratitude to each of you.

To all my family of origin from Argentina, and to my in-laws from Costa Rica. *Gracias*!

And, of course, to my immediate family: Erika, Matías Namdak, and Karina Dawa, a huge *gracias*! No words can fully express my love and gratitude to you, and how I relish all our moments together, including the many trips to be with the teachers mentioned here.

Thank you, *thugjeche*, *merci beaucoup*, and *mil gracias* to all of you!

CHAPTER ONE

An Introduction to Magical Movement

A Hidden Tradition

Downward dog, child's pose, warriors one, two, and three. Once a complete unknown, yoga has become so widespread in the West that you'd be hard-pressed to find someone who hasn't heard of it, and maybe even tried folding themselves, pretzel-like, into its positions at their local studio. In fact, downward dog and its ilk are so popular here that they've become almost synonymous with the word *yoga*.

In reality, these well-known poses come from a particular yogic tradition called hatha yoga, first brought to the West starting in the late 1800s and picking up steam midway through the 1900s. What many understand as yoga itself is actually just one particular branch of a much bigger tree of yogic traditions.

Another one of these branches, although still practiced to this day, is far less known in the West—*trulkhor*, or "magical movement," the yogic practices of Tibet. For a thousand years, Tibetan yoga has been part of Tibetan Buddhist spiritual training, used primarily to enhance meditation by clearing away mental and physical obstacles like anger or drowsiness. There are many kinds of magical movement practices in the different Tibetan traditions. All of the main traditions of Tibetan religion practice some kind of *trulkhor*, although it is most prevalent in the Kagyu and Nyingma schools of Buddhism as well as in Bön. I am blessed to have been practicing magical movements, first with the Nyingma and then with the Bön lineage, for almost thirty years.

The existence of Tibetan yoga may surprise even those familiar with Tibetan Bön and Buddhism, since Tibetan teachings in the West, until very recently, focused more on various mind-based practices such as concentration and visualization. For a long time, this lack of information gave magical movement an aura of secrecy or mysticism about it. Nowadays, though, magical movement is slowly being taught all over the world, and its instructional texts are being translated into English and other languages.

Yoga was one of the many spiritual practices that arose during the pan-Asian tantric movement, which began around the fourth century BCE and reached its apogee four hundred years later. Its wellspring may have been India, but it spread across Asia, mixing with local religious tradition and culture. While the exact history of the Tibetan tradition of magical movement has yet to be written, contemporary religious leaders and scholars date it back to at least the eighth century CE. Some even claim that different forms of it were practiced much earlier and preserved as an oral/aural tradition. Its existence can be definitively established by the eleventh century CE, so we can easily state that it has been practiced for at least a thousand years.

Why Practice Tibetan Yoga?

Although nowadays yoga is often understood as exercises that promote physical and mental health, at its core the purpose of all yoga is liberation—enlightenment—and traditionally defined, yogic practices are ones that make the body the locus and the tool for reaching enlightenment. So, like all traditional forms of yoga, enlightenment is the purpose of magical movement as well. In the Tibetan viewpoint it is a technique for enhancing meditation by getting rid of the mental and physical obstacles that block access to meditative states of mind. And, like many forms of yoga, it comes with its own wonderful nomenclature that reflect its culture of origin, meaning that if you follow this book's instructions, you may soon find yourself "striking the athlete's hammer" or moving as a "wild yak butting sideways."

For those less spiritually inclined, practicing magical movement also comes with a host of practical benefits. Traditionally, Tibetan yogis and accomplished meditators living in solitude in caves used it to help dispel all kinds of physical and mental illness. With no access to hospitals or any healthcare professionals, it was one of their only options for restoring good health, and by their accounts it served them well—so well that scientists have begun studying magical movement's health benefits, in particular for cancer patients, in randomized controlled trials. These benefits include stress reduction, the elimination of intrusive thoughts, and better sleep.

At this point, you may be wondering why I am specifically referring to Tibetan yoga as "magical movement." Why is it not simply called Tibetan yoga, the way that we say "hatha yoga" or refer to the well-known Tibetan devotional practice as "guru yoga"? The term used in the Tibetan texts, *trulkhor*, is a compound comprised of *trul* and *khor*. *Trul* is usually translated as "magic" or "magical." It can also take on the meaning of "machine" or "mechanics" when combined with *khor*, which literally means "wheel," but it can also be translated as "circular movement" or just "movement." Through many conversations with Ponlob Thinley Nyima, the current principal teacher at Menri Monastery in India and a magical movement master, we've settled together on "magical movement" as a translation, because of the magic-like experiences practicing this yoga generates.

I don't mean "magic" in the way that we usually understand it in the West, which might conjure images of wizards and wands. In Asian disciplines, magic has less to do with spells and charms and more to do with inner states of transformation. Lao Tzu, the writer of the *Dao De Jing*, wrote about practices that use the body to alter the mind: "It is internal transformation at the deepest level that becomes the most sought after religious experience. It is also a transformation often linked to magic."

This is the sense in which I am using the word *magic*. The magic that magical movement creates is inner transformation—inner magic. Tibetan yoga has the power to change the experience of the practitioner and their state of mind. In the old Tibetan texts, this could even mean the production of mystical experiences, like being able to walk without touching the ground or reversing the practitioner's age. Magical movement's healing properties, and its traditional consideration as medicine, can also be seen as "magical" in this way.

Or as Khenpo Tenpa Yungdrung, current abbot of Triten Norbutse Monastery in Nepal, says, the magic in "magical movement" refers to the "unusual effects that these movements produce in the experience of the practitioner." This is the magic of magical movement, and it's accessible to us all.

How the Magic Works

The Body-Breath-Mind Triad

Magical movement, like all yogas, is a "mind-body" practice, because it entails an understanding of the mind-body connection. This setup is different than the Western conception that often separates mind and body. In the yogic and Tibetan view, our mind is located in our body and affected by it, and vice-versa.

While Westerners often see the body as nothing more than its physical form—arms, legs, torso, and so on, with a subdermal system of interior organs and other physical networks—the Tibetan configuration conceives the body as a multi-layered dimension with components beyond just the physical ones. These invisible but experiential dimensions are sometimes referred to as the sacred anatomy or "subtle body." This subtle body is composed of a complex network of channels together with the winds that

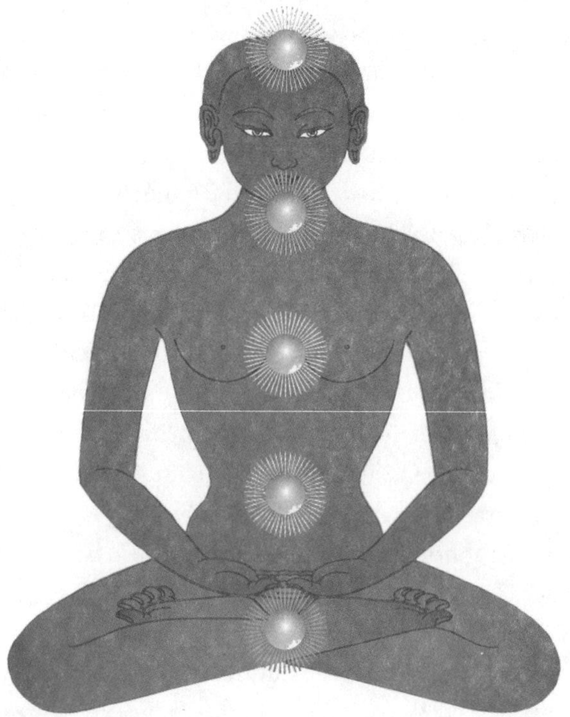

The five chakras of our subtle body

run within those channels. The subtle consciousness—our mind—rides through the body on these vital winds. The subtle body can thus be understood as the landscape where the mind and the physical body connect with each other. You are probably already familiar with the term chakras, which are the major junctures of these channels, places where immense vitality is gathered and also where obstructions to the vital winds occur.

In Tibetan spiritual traditions, body, energy (in this case breath-energy or wind), and mind are the three doors to enlightenment, meaning that they are the three loci of spiritual training. Magical movement integrates all three.

Among the thousands of meditative practices within the Tibetan traditions, while the three components of body, breath, and mind are always there, particular practices emphasize one over the others. The sitting meditation practices you're likely familiar with, for instance, in which the practitioner sits cross-legged in the lotus position, are a common method of emphasizing the mind over the body or breath. Of course, in the standard lotus pose for meditation the mind is supported by an unmoving body, and the breath is flowing naturally; the body and breath are involved, but are not being used as anything more than supports. But there are also many Tibetan practices that emphasize the body, like bowing or prostrations, circumambulation, pilgrimages, and of course, the yogic practices.

Different yogic traditions, while they all utilize the body as an aid for reaching enlightenment, have different techniques. In some Indian styles of yoga, the practitioner aims to hold a pose (*asana*), with the body unmoving and the breath flowing naturally. By keeping still in a specific body posture, the mind will stop and be stable. In other words, by controlling your body you control your mind.

In magical movement the practitioner actually holds the breath using a certain method—we'll get into this below—while the body moves. And in the particular magical movement lineage that we will be learning in this book, at the end of the movement the breath is released in a particular way, opening the possibility to reconnect to one's natural mind state. In magical movement the body and breath are not mere supports for a mind-focused practice, but are the main focus themselves. In this way magical movement is similar to Chinese mind-body practices such as tai chi and qigong, which share with Tibetan yoga the aspect of developing focused attention through movement. In contrast to magical movement, though, in tai chi and qigong the breath is not held but rather maintained as naturally as possible, more like in Indian yogas.

We'll get more into the specifics as we go on, but for now, remember that magical movement brings a different conception of the body to the foreground, that of the internal landscapes of the sacred anatomy or subtle body and its dynamics. This subtle body is the place of all yogic training, including magical movement, which integrates the body, the breath, and the mind on the way to liberation.

Clearing Away Obstacles

It is also at the level of the subtle body that magical movement works its magic, so to speak—the removal of physical and mental obstacles that are blocking desired mental states. This is a common feature in Tibetan yogic traditions. In Tibetan, the term used is *geksel*, literally "clearing (*sel*) away the obstacles (*gek*)." In simpler language, the great Bön teacher Yongdzin Tenzin Namdak says that magical movement should be used when one's meditation state is unclear, unstable, or weakened in some way, because magical movement will clear out whatever is causing the issue and help one to reconnect to the natural state of mind. You can think of it like a reboot that sweeps away any bugs in the system.

Ponlob Thinley Nyima believes that each magical movement technique was created when a practitioner needed to overcome an obstacle to meditation and found through experience that a particular movement helped. So, specific magical movements tackle specific things. For example, "rolling the four limbs like wheels" is helpful for overcoming pride; "waving the silk tassel upward" helps overcome jealousy; and "stance of a tigress's leap" overcomes drowsiness and agitation. There are also sets that focus on specific areas of the body.

Obstacles are removed in the landscape of the subtle body—the channels it's composed of, the breath currents or winds that run through those channels, and the mind that rides on that breath. Magical movement is based on what is known as *tsalung*, the practices of the channels (*tsa*) and winds (*lung*). In these, the practitioner becomes familiar with the channels of the subtle body first through visualization and then by using the mind to direct the breath and winds along those channels. In this way, the wind is made to circulate through the channels more evenly in terms of the rhythm of the inhalation and exhalation, and with a greater balance in terms of the amount and strength of the winds through the different channels.

The mind rides on the wind, like a rider on a horse, and the two travel together through the pathways of the channels. As the wind circulating in the channels becomes more even and balanced, the channels turn increasingly pliable, allowing the winds to find their own comfortably smooth rhythm. When the wind rhythm is smooth, like a wave, the mind riding on it has a smoother ride, too, which reduces agitation.

With the help of movements that guide the mind and the winds into different areas of the body, magical movement brings forth the possibility of healing or harmonizing the entire body-energy-mind system. This kind of harmony is a short-term goal of all yogic practices (the ultimate goal, remember, is enlightenment) and is also a model of good health that is in line with the concept of well-being in Tibetan medicine. In magical movement in particular, the releasing of specific obstacles using specific movements allows the winds to flow better throughout. Rather than a "tin man," whose being is obstructed by various broken-down parts, your whole ecosystem of body, breath/wind, and mind becomes like a well-oiled machine.

As you become more familiar with magical movement, you become more familiar with your breath entering through your nostrils into your channels and also more sensitive to the subtler winds. Smaller and more distinctive winds start to open up, thus generating experiences that support spiritual practice or alter those that are detrimental—in other words, the magic.

A last crucial point: it's not just you who is being changed by the magic. As in all Tibetan spiritual practices, magical movement is practiced with the motivation that the ultimate goal of enlightenment is for the benefit of every conscious entity in the entire universe—what the tradition calls "all sentient beings." In Tibetan tantric practices the body is perceived as an inner mandala, a sacred space of our inner universe that can be affected by contemplative practices. As the practitioner purifies the inner mandala, they affect and are affected by the external mandala: the world and the beings in it.

In more down-to-earth terms, contemporary magical movement teachers emphasize that a practitioner should integrate their meditative experiences into their daily life, creating a ripple effect from the meditation mat to everyday life. As we train and calm our minds, guiding and focusing our breath, our thoughts, speech, and actions become less reactive and more present and compassionate. The idea is that meaningful change begins with ourselves.

Abiding in the Natural State of Mind

The purpose of clearing obstacles is to enhance the meditative state. Because magical movement unblocks and opens the flow of the winds, magical movement serves as a gateway to a more clear, open, and stable experience of abiding in the natural state of mind. The "natural state of mind" will be familiar to anyone who has practiced in the Dzogchen tradition, the tradition of Tibetan teachings that exists primarily in the Nyingma and Bön schools.

In the Dzogchen tradition, the natural state of mind is that in which the mind is clear, blissful, and free of conceptual noise. The Dzogchen teachings say that all sentient beings have as their birthright this pristine inner state, a concept known as "buddha nature." But because that state is veiled by all kinds of obstacles—all of the human behavior and mental activity that we are used to and which cause manifold agitation—one needs to discover, "see," or experience it. It is like a jewel covered in mud, or glass of water full of swirling silt. There are many practices in the Dzogchen tradition aimed at revealing and then maintaining the experience of the natural state of mind. Magical movement is one of them. Magical movement, then, is a way to connect to our buddha nature, to our latent wisdom or insight, with the mediating structure being the subtle body.

While magical movement, as I've said, is practiced across all Tibetan religious traditions, there are differences between them. This book presents the particular lineage of magical movement that I've personally studied and practiced for thirty years. This is magical movement as presented in the Bön

Dzogchen treatise titled *Zhang Zhung Aural Transmission* (hereafter we'll call it the *ZZ Aural Transmission* for ease). The text's chapter on magical movement is called *Quintessential Oral Instructions*.

According to traditional accounts, the *ZZ Aural Transmission* was first taught in the eighth century. However, I would date *Quintessential Oral Instructions* to around the late eleventh or early twelfth century, since the names of the masters mentioned in that chapter include some from the eleventh century. This chapter, along with the thirteenth-century magical movement chapter in *Experiential Transmission* by Drugyalwa Yungdrung and the early twentieth-century *Commentary* by Shardza Tashi Gyaltsen, are the main sources of these magical movement teachings for present-day Bön practitioners, both laypersons and monastics. In the discussion below I will base my discussion of the magical movements on the instructions given in all three texts.

In the *ZZ Aural Transmission* lineage, as mentioned above, one performs the physical movements—we'll go through these together—while at the same time holding the breath in a "neutral way," which I'll explain in more detail below. Holding the breath in this manner during each exercise allows the wind to pervade throughout the body, and so I will refer to the method as a neutral holding to connect to one's "pervasive wind." This means it is also available to aid the practitioner in residing or resting in the natural state of mind.

Every movement ends with shaking one's four limbs and an exhalation accompanied by the sounds of *ha* and *phat*—these are two common vocalizations in Tibetan practices, although they aren't usually used together. The shaking arms and legs help stir inner obstacles, and the exhalation and the vocalizations both help to cut through mental noise and expel obstacles, so you can remain more completely in the natural state of mind. It's like a dam holding back a river. Holding the breath creates pressure, and energy builds up. With the exhale and exclamation, the dam is removed and the river is released. The torrent of water sweeps away what's in its path. For a moment or more, you experience the natural state of mind flowing like a pristine river, its waters clear. Or you feel that you can remain fully present with the support of a vast, clear sky.

Making Magic Together

As in many yogic traditions, knowing that there is a lineage of teachings that has continued, unbroken, from master to disciple, teacher to student, is very important. This is as true in the Bön tradition I study, with its lineage of teachers, as well as the texts, commentaries, and the living teachers, as it is also in the Buddhist traditions of Tibet.

Bön is a native Tibetan tradition that finds its roots in earliest Tibetan history, long before Buddhism arrived from India and China. Over the centuries it has shared many of its characteristics and practices with Buddhist traditions, and it has in turn absorbed much from Buddhism, including terminology and many outward elements of appearance—so much so that it's often difficult for the nonspecialist to distinguish between a Bön and a Buddhist community. The scriptures, doctrine, and practices of the tradition were only formally organized during the Tibetan Renaissance of the eleventh and twelfth centuries, the period in which the Buddhist traditions as they are known today were also first organized, systematizing long-standing oral traditions such as magical movement.

The Bön tradition ascribes the development of the magical movement practices described in this book to a handful of yogins who are themselves shrouded in mystery. All three of our source texts—the eleventh-century *Quintessential Oral Instructions*, the thirteenth-century *Experiential Transmission* by Drugyalwa, and the twentieth-century *Commentary* by Shardza—agree on the names of lineages masters who composed the magical movement cycles first written down in the *ZZ Aural Transmission*. Drugyalwa's colophon is representative:

> This successive root, branch, and distinctive magical movements all flow from the *Zhang Zhung Aural Transmission*. The lineage began with Pongyal Tsenpo, the first of the six destroyers of delusion, also called the masters of the upper tradition. He passed it to the five great accomplished masters of the lower tradition, and then on to Yangton Chenpo and his lineage of the northern and southern traditions, from whence it came to me, Drugyalwa Yungdrung.

Some of these members of these two groupings, the "masters of the upper and lower traditions"—of the western Tibetan regions of Dolpo and the Kailash area, and Kham and Amdo, respectively—coexisted in the same historical period, making the exact chronology difficult to chart. (The lineages known as the northern and southern traditions branched off from Bumje Ö, the teacher credited with writing *Quintessential Oral Instructions*.)

This magical movement lineage thus begins with Pongyal Tsenpo, whom all our texts mention as the first teacher of the magical movement sets in the form they now exist. According to Samten Karmay in his book *Little Luminous Boy*, prior to Pongyal Tsenpo the magical movement teachings were passed down orally from a master to a single disciple. Pongyal Tsenpo was the first to teach more than one student: he transmitted the oral tradition to a disciple named Lhundrub Muthur and initiated the written tradition by writing it down and passing it to Sherab Loden.

Pongyal Tsenpo also taught Togme Shigpo, whom the *ZZ Aural Transmission* names as the sixth member of the "destroyers of delusion," or the masters of the upper tradition, and the second in our lineage. Third was Lhundrub Muthur, who, as noted above, was also a student of Pongyal Tsenpo, and fourth was Orgom Kundul. Lhundrub Muthur and Orgom Kundrul are also identified as the first and fifth members of the masters of the lower tradition, respectively. Togme Shigpo and Orgom Kundul both taught Yangton Chenpo, who thereby reunited the oral and written traditions. He passed them on to his wife, Nyanmo Tashi Jochan, and together they taught their son Bumje Ö, who wrote them down in the *ZZ Aural Transmission*, most likely in the eleventh century. Yangton Chenpo and his son Bumje Ö, the last two masters mentioned in the magical movement lineage, were part of the famous Dzogchen Yangton lineage, which later moved to what is now the Dolpo region of northwest Nepal. Ponlob Thinley Nyima is from this region and is a contemporary master of this lineage. As we will see below, the teachers named in the lineage are each credited with the development of different sets of magical movements.

Magical movement reached a pinnacle in thirteenth-century Tibet, likely the result of the Tibetan Renaissance, when the body resurged as a center of attention for spiritual practice. It was during this period that Drugyalwa composed his *Experiential Transmission*. From there, however, we jump straight into the modern period. I have not been able to find any texts or commentaries on magical movement that date from between the fourteenth and the nineteenth centuries. There seem to be no developments in magical movement between Drugyalwa and its revival by Shardza Tashi Gyaltsen four hundred years later.

Shardza, the author of the *Commentary* on which this book is based, was one of the most widely recognized Bönpo lamas of recent times. He studied the magical movement teachings of both the *ZZ Aural Transmission* and of another critical text, *Instructions on the A.* Using these, he designed a one-hundred-day practice retreat curriculum for magical movement, which is in his *Main Points*. This significant contribution to systematizing and clarifying the teachings has made it much easier to practice magical movement and has ensured its survival into the present-day; his curriculum is how magical movement is practiced today in the main Bön monasteries, both inside Tibet and in exile.

Moving Forward

However, magical movement has also been lost in many places where it used to flourish, and it has been slow to disseminate outside of Tibetan communities. As mentioned above, most of the physical yogas that are taught in the West come from the Hindu traditions. When Westerners began receiving Tibetan teachings, these were mainly meditative-focused ways to develop the mind. I think this was due to two reasons: The first is that Western practitioners of Tibetan Buddhism felt that the mind practices were more important, and thus asked lamas only for mind-related teachings. The second is that many of the lamas themselves supported this view and were either not trained in magical movement or felt that it could lead to problems for the practitioners if not sufficiently supervised. Thus, there has been a long-term drought of information about magical movement.

Nevertheless, nearly a century after Shardza composed his *Commentary*, there seems to be a growing interest in the West in the Tibetan physical yoga techniques, and they are now being taught in the US, Latin America, and Europe. For example, one can study them at Namkhai Norbu Rinpoche's

Dzogchen community and also at Tenzin Wangyal Rinpoche's Ligmincha International, which offers special magical movement retreats. And in the last few years alone, *Yoga Journal* published three articles on Tibetan yoga: one on the different types of Tibetan yogas that have come to the US; a second one on the magical movement paintings of the "*naga* temple," also known as the secret temple of the Dalai Lamas in Lhasa, Tibet; and one on the benefits of magical movement with cancer patients.

This last topic, the intersection of Western and Tibetan medicine, has been one I have been especially excited to be a part of. Mainstream Western medicine has long failed to recognize the connection between physical illness and energetic or mental obstacles. Now there are new paradigms that include the bio-psycho-social-spiritual model in the emerging field of Complementary and Integrative Medicine (CIM) that are more akin to Asian medical systems. Beginning in the 1930s and flourishing especially from the 1970s onward, and with more scientific interest from the 1990s until today, there have been thousands of studies of meditation reported in journals and books, and many graduate theses and dissertations written on the possible benefits of mind-body practices in different populations.

In 1999, after a year of facilitating Tibetan meditation at The Place of Wellness (now the Integrative Medicine Center) at the University of Texas MD Anderson Cancer Center, Lorenzo Cohen, a behavioral researcher there, asked me to propose a research "intervention" based on Tibetan mind-body practices. With support and interest from Yongdzin Tenzin Namdak and Tenzin Wangyal Rinpoche, who became an advisor to the research, we formed an MD Anderson–Ligmincha International team, scientifically led by Dr. Cohen, with the aim of investigating the possible effects of a Tibetan yoga intervention for people with cancer.

Since then, we have put together a number of studies: one with lymphoma patients, a few with women with breast cancer, and one with lung cancer patients and their caregivers. Participants in the lymphoma study, which tracked behavioral changes, reported improved sleep, including longer duration, less use of sleep medications, and better sleep quality, as well as greater ease getting to sleep. (Improving sleep quality in a cancer population may be particularly salient as sleep is crucial for recovery, and fatigue and sleep disturbances are common side effects of cancer.)

This outcome brought positive attention to our studies, and we received funding from the National Institute of Health's National Cancer Institute for a larger study for women with breast cancer undergoing chemotherapy. One of the results we saw in that study was the necessary "dose" of magical movement. Only those who practiced more than twice a week were able to tap into and maintain the benefits of the Tibetan yoga program.

This research, I feel, is in its infancy—or maybe puberty, at best. These randomized controlled trials are among the growing number of studies of yoga in cancer patient populations; it is interesting to remember that our lymphoma pilot study was the first published scientific yoga study in any cancer population, and the first scientific study of magical movement in any population. This points to a future rife with possibilities—like eventually tracking magical movement's effect on other populations or general disease progression—and magical movement is part of the playground for an inclusive dialogue between Western medicine and the ancient yogic disciplines.

Wherever that future leads, so far it has been startling and moving to watch magical movement travel from Tibet to India and Nepal, and now to the world; from transmission between Tibetan masters and disciples to being taught to cancer patients in Texas. Much of magical movement's history has yet to be written, but it is clear that its next chapter will be a rich one. Just by reading this book, you are now an integral part of the story, too. The magic has been released. Let's see what it can do.

✧ CHAPTER TWO ✧

How the Magic Works

The center of the victorious mandala, one's own body
The source of all positive qualities without exception
Is the expanse of the three channels and the five chakras
I take I refuge in this body of emptiness.
—Tenzin Wangyal Rinpoche

Preparing for Magic: Channels, Winds, and Magical Movement

Understanding the subtle body and its elements is crucial to the effectiveness of magical movement. The Bön tradition teaches the importance of preparing for practice by purifying the channels and the winds, which one begins with a simple technique of expelling and inhaling air through the nostrils and guiding the winds through the channels.

This is a method for the practitioner to expel any poisons associated with the winds and train their body's subtle channels. One should forcefully expel the coarse breath through the right nostril and then leisurely inhale long gentle breath through the left nostril. Through this simple practice, the practitioner becomes familiar with their subtle body, gaining the capacity to fully engage in more advanced practices. It is through the training of the winds that the practitioner learns to guide the breath via the channels. With powerful exhalations and nurturing inhalations, the practitioner clears away the obstacles that are the poisons that impede the flow of the winds. And one comes to perceive that the channels are paths for both the winds and the mind, which together flow like a horse and rider.

What kinds of obstacles can you expect to encounter when you begin this practice? When the mind is distracted by one of the afflictions, when the wind

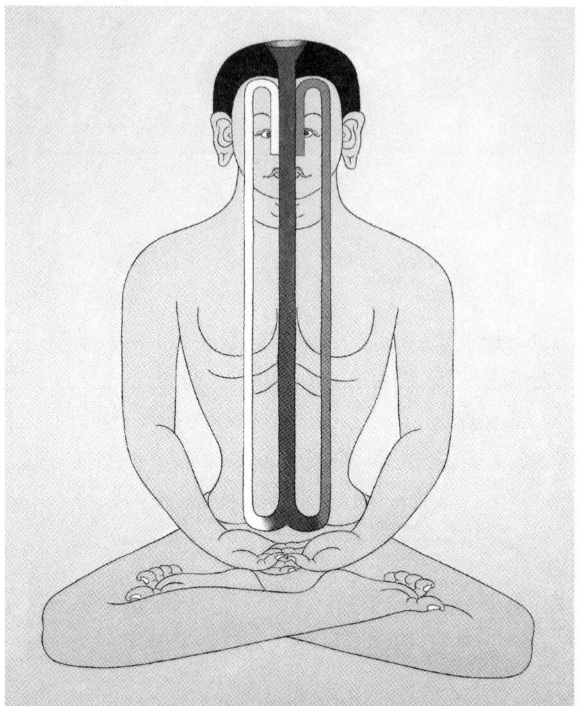

The three main channels of the subtle body

is interrupted by an illness, or when there are spirit-provoked obstacles—a rich category of obstacles in the traditional Tibetan world view—the wind cannot flow through the channels in the proper way, and the mind is therefore obstructed. This is why rooting out the poisons is so important.

Having thereby cleansed the channels, the practitioner then trains in manipulating the breath by holding it in a specific way. In all the subsequent training of the winds, the practitioner needs to implement what is known as the *neutral wind*, which we will refer to as "neutral holding." In his *Commentary*, Shardza emphasizes that neutral holding, which allows the wind to pervade the entire body, is employed in *every* magical movement. This neutral holding needs to be developed in three ways: (1) the gentle holding of the wind, (2) the intermediate holding of the wind, and (3) the strong holding of the wind, or forceful wind. The first is likened to a basket, the second is likened to a vase, and the last is called a mass of fire, or fireball. All three of these are done in four sessions in which you inhale and exhale 108 times. A trained instructor can

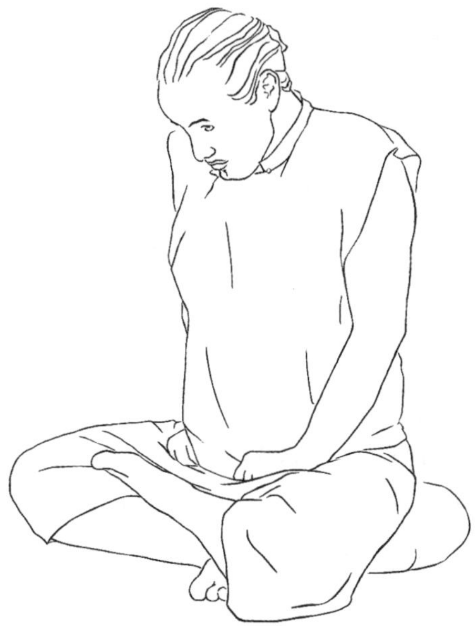

Posture for developing gentle, intermediate, and forceful wind

guide you on mastering this technique; it is enough for beginners to hold the breath with the intention of pervading it throughout the body.

These two steps represent the initial practices, and from here one can proceed to perform the magical movements.

What follows below is a very simple introduction to the thirty-nine separate movements in the sequence as laid out in our source texts. These are divided into four basic categories, three of which are further divided into two parts: (1) foundational movements, (2) root movements and root movements that clear away obstacles, (3) branch movements and branch movements that clear away obstacles, and (4) distinctive movements that clear away specific obstacles and distinctive movements that clear away common obstacles.

Foundational Magical Movements

The first set of magical movements is known as the "foundational magical movements," a cycle that consists of five separate movements. According to Shardza, *Quintessential Oral Instructions* detailed six, but through oral explanations these are condensed into the following five:

1. Purification of the Head
2. Purification of the Legs
3. Purification of the Arms
4. Purification of the Upper Torso
5. Purification of the Lower Part of the Body

Some contemporary teachers, such as Ponlob Thinley Nyima, maintain the regime of six from *Quintessential Oral Instructions*, explaining that practitioners should do a combination of all six parts (head, right arm, left arm, right leg, left leg, and upper body) as one single magical movement in the style of an "energetic massage." However, in reinterpreting this foundational magical movement of six parts from *Quintessential Oral Instructions* and crafting the five individual magical movements that he describes in the *Commentary*, Shardza brings clearer meaning to us as practitioners. I will thus follow Shardza's presentation of five foundational magical movements. In practice and teaching I would do both the "energetic massage" of six parts from *Quintessential Oral Instructions* followed by Shardza's five individual magical movements.

This initial cycle is designed to purify obstacles of different parts of the body, with a succession of purificatory massage-like magical movements. Having previously done the preparation of the subtle body through the training of the channels and winds described above, the practitioner now works on the physical body as a tool toward purification.

We begin by taking the well-known cross-legged meditation known as *yungdrung*. (Note that *yungdrung* in Tibetan—swastika in Sanskrit—is an ancient Asian religious symbol of prosperity and good fortune. It also symbolizes, like the *dorje* or *vajra*, indestructibility and eternity.) This five-point meditation posture can sometimes mean full lotus (legs totally crossed, ankles resting on opposite thighs) or half lotus (one leg on top of the other). The different elements of the posture are said to produce distinct benefits:

- Supporting the generation of heat by having the legs crossed into one's body.

- Allowing the winds to flow smoothly through the body by keeping the spine straight.
- Maintaining alertness by keeping the chest open "like an eagle soaring in the sky."
- Reducing discursive thoughts by keeping the neck slightly bent forward.
- Generating bliss by keeping the mind clear through gazing with one's eyes slightly open, looking naturally forward and keeping the hands in the position of equipoise: resting comfortably, palms upward on the lap, left upon right, about four finger widths below the navel.

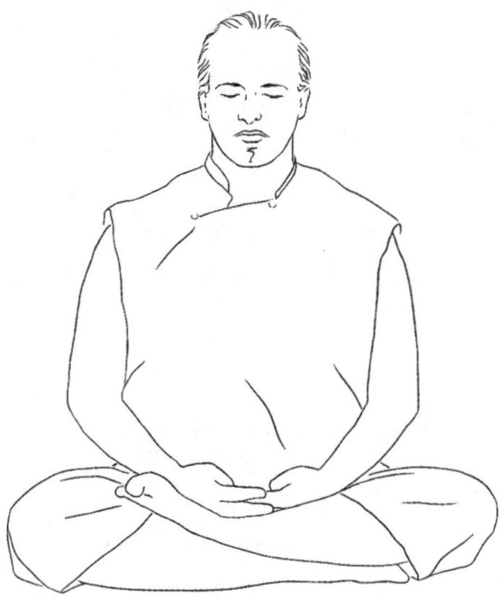

Five-point meditation posture

Purification of the Head

In this posture, with the breath held in the neutral way, one begins by vigorously rubbing one's hands above one's head until the hands have become warm. With the hands heated, one sweeps downwardly along the right, left, and front of the head in order to help direct the pervasive wind and clear away any obstacles of the head. As one feels contact with one's obstacles, be it physical illnesses, emotional or mental obstructions, or a spirit's provocations, one sweeps away the obstacles with the winds that guide them out. The movement ends with the shaking of the four limbs, expelling sounds and visualization, which brings in the other two parts of one's being, the breath and the mind. Shardza instructs:

> In order to expel illnesses, demons, negativities, and obscurations, sound *ha* and shake cyclic existence from its depths by shaking the body and limbs; while reflecting that all sentient beings are buddhas, pronounce the sound *phat*: apply these two practices to all the magical movements.

The combination of the physical posture, the mind's support in the task of clearing, and the guidance of the winds has the power to release external, internal, and secret obstacles, not just for oneself but for all sentient beings. This is part of the magic that allows the practitioner to be able to connect to one's natural state of mind—to emerge from the "depths of cyclic existence" to a state of primordial purity. This can be called the inner magic or the mystical effect of the practice. Shardza adds, "these vocalizations should be applied to all the magical movements."

About Breathing, Shaking, and Concluding with Ha *and* Phat

It is worth pausing here to reiterate the importance of the breathing process that applies to all the magical movements. The wind is pervasive—it fills the entire body—and it is activated through neutral holding. Inhaling from the side channels into the central channel, with neutral holding, allows the wind to reach where the three channels unite—located four finger widths below the navel. From there it spreads up the central channel and throughout the body like sun rays. This is the process that I will call the mandala dynamic. That dynamic is the same in all movements; however, the movements themselves define not only the external shape but also the way the winds are guided, and thus the mandalic display (externally and internally) varies from movement to movement. The state of mind accessed should be the same, but the sensations that color that experience may differ. I will mention some examples of this as I describe other magical movements.

The combined *ha* and *phat* vocalization, which is another vital aspect of each magical movement, is unique to Bön. Some Buddhist magical movement texts, such as the Nyingma *Union of Sun and Moon*, describe exhalations with *ha*, alone. Other meditative practices use either *ha* or *phat*, but to my knowledge none combine the two in this way. Although some sections of *Quintessential Oral Instructions* mention only *ha* for the concluding exhalation, it is clear from other sections that *ha* and *phat* are both applied to all magical movements, and Shardza's *Commentary* further reaffirms that both *ha* and *phat* are used in the concluding sections.

Shardza explains that this vocalization of *ha* and *phat* is done together with the shaking of the four limbs, which draws forth the internal obstacles. As he puts it, *ha* is used "in order to expel illnesses, demons, negativities, and obscurations," and *phat* to "shake cyclic existence from its depth by shaking the body and limbs while reflecting that all sentient beings are buddhas." That is, one shakes one's body to call forth all the suffering of all beings and the causes of that suffering, and to prepare to clear them all. Thus the shaking is performed with the thought that one is in fact shaking all obstacles from the depth of samsara—that is, all the suffering of all sentient beings—in order to liberate them together with oneself. Then, with the vocalizations, one exhales and cleans those obstacles away, remaining in a clearer state of mind, or, more precisely, in a clearer mind-energy-body system, where one feels that all beings and oneself are beings of light in a luminous mandala: a Buddha mandala, source of all positive qualities without exception.

The magical movements that follow in the foundational set are the purification of the legs, the arms, the torso, and the lower part of the body. All of them are performed seated, with the conclusion done either seated or standing up. One concludes with the shaking of the four limbs, the vocalizations, and the visualization as beings of light, or buddhas, as described above. After performing each magical movement and its concluding shaking and vocalization, the lamas advise to "stay in that experience until it loses its freshness." This means that you can strive to remain in that pure experience, and when the experience of a relaxed and clear state of mind begins to fade, it is time to perform the next magical movement. Thus, after the purification of the head, remain for a moment in a centered, relaxed, and clear state of mind, energy, and body, and after a few moments, begin the next magical movement.

Purification of the Legs

Seated with legs extended to the front and parallel to each other, one is instructed to inhale, with neutral holding, allowing the pervasive wind to be guided by one hand through each leg in turn as if it were an energetic massage. One's right hand sweeps slightly above the right leg or lightly touches the leg, starting at the waist and proceeding toward the feet. The downward sweeping movement purifies all obstacles in the leg. As the hand reaches the foot, one is instructed to grab the toes and raise the leg upward, shaking slightly, and then let the leg go down to the ground again. This movement is repeated seven times. Then, repeat with the left hand on the left leg, also seven times. One concludes with the shaking, shuddering, visualization, and vocalizations as explained earlier.

Purification of the Arms

Seated in the cross-legged posture, one is instructed to create a special hand gesture, or *mudra*, called diamond-scepter, *dorje*, or *vajra* fist. This powerful gesture is frequently employed in both Bön and Buddhism. In this case, though, instead of having the thumb tucked inside the fist at the base of the ring finger, the thumb emerges slightly between the middle and ring fingers, pressing against the ring finger. Noteworthy is that constricting the ring finger in both these forms of the gesture is a common Tibetan way of preventing spirits from entering and disturbing one's energetic system.

One extends the right arm sideways, bringing it back to the armpit seven times, and then does the same with the left. The point in the armpit where the fist touches is said to be an especially energetic point, believed to enhance the experience of clarity. As the arm extends, one feels the winds run through that arm and sweep obstacles from it. Instead of having the arms and hands sweep away obstacles as with the two preceding movements, here it is through a strong sideways movement that each arm purifies itself. One concludes with the same shaking, stirring, visualization, exhalation, and vocalization as usual, remaining in the experience as long as it is clear.

Purification of the Upper Torso

The upper torso is purified next. In *yungdrung*, or cross-legged posture, one sits erect, which straightens the torso and helps align the channels in a straight position. This allows the clearest flow of the wind in the torso area. Extending both arms in front and drawing them inward, one touches or slightly pounds the chest area with the heel of the hand seven times. At the end, after the shaking the limbs and the exhalation, the vocalization in this movement is *ha*, *ha*, *ha*, *phat*. This is the only movement in which one is instructed to exhale with three *ha*'s instead of one. Also, it is the only one within this set in which the area purified is not massaged or lightly touched, but pounded. The purification is effected through that triple exhalation; the *ha*'s themselves expel what the thumping in the torso frees. After discussions with different lamas, I infer that the three consecutive *ha*'s are associated with the release of the three kinds of obstacles mentioned earlier: external, internal, and secret.

Purification of the Lower Body

For the last movement in this set one begins in the same posture as in the purification of the legs: one is seated with both legs extended in front and parallel to each other. However, here, after inhaling and holding the breath in the usual neutral way, one raises one's hands above the head before bringing them down together, first making contact at the waist and then sweeping them down along both legs, like an energetic massage brushing obstacles away. Reaching the toes, one extends the arms and legs and shakes all four limbs slightly, feeling that some of the subtler obstacles are freed through the fingers and toes, all the while maintaining the hold with pervasive wind. One repeats this movement seven times and then concludes as with the other magical movements, with *ha* and *phat*.

Benefits of the Foundational Magical Movements

It is common with many Tibetan texts on esoteric practices that the benefits of a practice are usually articulated after the instructions are completed. The benefits of the five foundational magical movements are described as follows in the *Commentary*, itself based on *Quintessential Oral Instructions*:

> The foundational magical movements balance the channels and winds, clearing the interior of the channels. The four elements are balanced, and the vital points of the aggregates of the body are penetrated, making the body function well. Awareness is lucid and the flow of each of the distinct winds is freed.

One could say that each of the movements of this set, understood by tradition to have been first compiled by Pongyal Tsenpo and ultimately redesigned by Shardza Tashi Gyaltsen, helps the practitioner release external, internal, and secret obstacles of the whole body. These obstacles could be understood as interruptions to one's connection to the nature of the mind. Or, and not necessarily incompatible with the former, these obstacles can be viewed as provoking numerous physical, energetic, and mental disturbances. The texts also emphasize that having cleared the channels of its obstructions, the channels and the winds that circulate through them are put under control. This, in turn, balances the four elements (air, fire, water, and earth—and space, when five elements are used), making the whole organism function harmoniously. With one's body established as a cleansed receptacle, and the subtle winds flowing unobstructedly, the mind's awareness gains lucidity. In simple terms, as the channels open up and the winds open up, they circulate better. Thus, one becomes purer, and wisdom increases.

It is important for the practitioner to remember at the end of each magical movement to perform the shaking of the four limbs. This internally stirs all the afflictions, obstacles, and obscurations not just of oneself but also of all beings in cyclic existence, which are then expelled. That focus of the mind, together with the strong exhalation with the sounds of *ha* and *phat*, allows the practitioner to release all those obstacles and connect to an undefiled state. This is what one tries to maintain as long as the experience remains fresh. Only after the experience fades does one continue with the next magical movement. One could think of this process as pouring clean water in a dirty bottle, stirring it, and pouring the water back out. The more one does this, the cleaner the bottle will become. Our body-energy-mind system is currently defiled, like pure water mixed with dirt. The more magical movements we do, the fewer the obscurations become, until our natural state is revealed. One could say that there is a cumulative effect in performing the magical movements in terms of cleansing, and also in terms of helping one to become more familiar and more settled with the natural state of mind.

Root Magical Movements

The root cycle is composed of two sets: the primary root itself, which has six magical movements, and the six magical movements that dispel obsta-

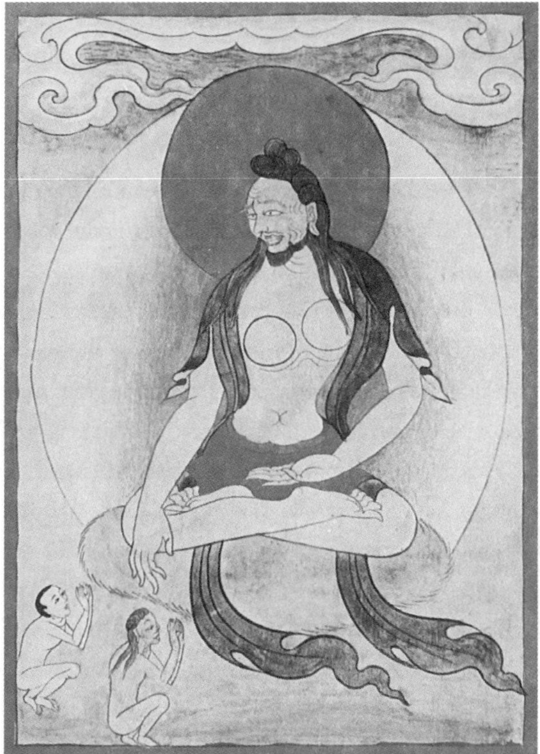

Pongyal Tsenpo

cles. In *Quintessential Oral Instructions* there are six primary root, or "root of the root," magical movements and only five magical movements that dispel obstacles, but Shardza adds a sixth in the *Commentary*. As we will see below, the five—an important number in both Bön and Buddhism—are made to correspond to five different sets of doctrinal categories: the poisons, the aggregates, the elements, the wisdoms, and the buddha dimensions. These correspondences will be explained in the benefits section below. When there is a sixth, it can be understood as a combination of the five, or a particular quality that helps complete the five, as we will see below.

The six primary root magical movements are:

1. Striking the Athlete's Hammer to Overcome Anger
2. The Skylight of Primordial Wisdom to Overcome Delusion
3. Rolling the Four Limbs like Wheels to Overcome Pride
4. Loosening the Corner of the Braided Knot to Overcome Attachment
5. Waving the Silk Tassel Upward to Overcome Jealousy
6. The Stance of a Tigress's Leap to Overcome Drowsiness and Agitation

Each magical movement in this set aims at overcoming or appeasing one of the five principal obstructive afflictions or poisons: anger, delusion, pride, attachment, and jealousy. The last of these, "the stance of a tigress's leap," overcomes the two main obstructions to a stable, meditative state of mind: drowsiness and agitation. Their names evoke the way the body will move in order to achieve each goal, maintaining the wind flowing in the pneumatic mandala-dynamic way, and allowing the mind to settle in its own natural state. According to Tenzin Wangyal Rinpoche, this set is the most important for a practitioner to learn and practice. In each magical movement the full movement is repeated seven times; in some this involves seven times on each side. The breath is held for the entire movement and only released when all repetitions are complete. At that point the practitioner concludes with the shaking, visualizations, and vocalizations of *ha* and *phat* as explained earlier.

Striking the Athlete's Hammer to Overcome Anger

For the "striking the athlete's hammer" movement one begins by standing on one's knees, with the back straight, the legs crossed behind at the ankles, and the hands interlaced behind one's neck. Keeping this posture, one bends forward from the waist, touching both elbows to the knees—left elbow to left knee, right elbow to right knee—and then returns to the initial posture. Holding one's breath as usual, one repeats this movement in a flowing motion seven times.

One's body takes the shape and action of hammer; by holding the neck with both hands one brings the hammer down and back as one bends to the front and comes up again. One can imagine that anger itself is being struck from one's being, or alternately, that simply by the exhaustion from the movement anger dissipates. Internally, as one inhales and rises into this posture, the wind works particularly in the chest area, opening up any blockages or constrictions. Furthermore, as we will see in the benefits section below, this movement relates to the element of space. Thus, in the initial position of keeping the back straight and chest area open—to which one returns with each repetition—the anger seems to be dissolved within space.

The Skylight of Primordial Wisdom to Overcome Delusion

In the "skylight of primordial wisdom" movement, one takes the cross-legged posture—preferably full lotus posture—with both hands on the hips and the elbows on the knees. The arms are bent to form two triangular windows or skylights. Gently rock back and forth, such that the head reaches toward the ground—ideally the nape of the neck would touch the ground when rolling backward, and the forehead when rocking forward. As one moves forward and backward, maintaining the "skylight" with one's arms, the heaviness of mental fogginess is said to dissipate like smoke through an open window.

Rolling the Four Limbs like Wheels to Overcome Pride

In this movement, "rolling the four limbs," which can take a bit of practice to master, once again take the cross-legged posture, keeping the torso straight and open, arms reaching to grab the toes with one's hands—right hand to left foot, left hand to right foot. One first leans back in that posture and then swings forward and rises to one's knees, keeping the body upright like a vertical stroke of a pen or brush, before swinging back again. As one repeats this seven times, the body rolling like a wheel back and forth, the four radiant wheels, or chakras, of the crown, throat, heart, and navel also spin. As these open, the sense of stiffness, sometimes associated with pride and haughtiness, is slowly softened and eventually overcome.

Loosening the Corner of the Braided Knot to Overcome Attachment

For "loosening the corner braided knot" one sits in the cross-legged posture, with the elbows extended to the side and the thumbs hooked under the armpits, the other fingers pointing toward the heart chakra, in the middle of the chest. As one performs this movement one feels like one is loosening a braided knot. The "knot" is the manifestation of desire or attachment; by liberating the braided knot, one can liberate one's attachments. This is done by bringing the elbows to the opposite knees seven times—starting with your right elbow to your left knee—alternating between the two and returning to center in between. Externally this eases stiffness as internally it liberates attachment.

Waving the Silk Tassel Upward to Overcome Jealousy

The magical movement called "waving the silk tassel upward" is done to overcome the poison of jealousy. Planting the left foot and hand on the ground, with the torso and leg extended and the arm firm, the right leg and arm are waved skyward seven times. One then repeats the movement seven times on the other side. In this magical movement, as one's body weight inclines to one side, supported by the leg and arm, the other side feels free, with the free arm and leg waving harmoniously upward like a silk tassel in the wind. This fluttering movement is felt not just in the arm and leg but also in the entire body, especially the lower back, and helps to release the internal tightness of jealousy.

The Stance of a Tigress's Leap to Overcome Drowsiness and Agitation

The sixth magical movement of the root set is an active engagement of the whole body. One begins by standing and bending forward, passing both hands behind one's legs and reaching to touch one's ears—if one cannot reach the ears, touching one's chin or as close to the face as possible is accepted. Maintaining this position, one hops seven times forward and seven times backward. On many occasions I have seen practitioners laugh as they try to engage in this posture; it is far from easy, but quite amusing. With perseverance, however, as one maintains the posture and performs the movement, all obstacles of drowsiness and agitation can be released. One feels awakened by the active exhausting engagement of the pose. In other words, one feels reinvigorated, having overcome the hindering tendencies of drowsiness and agitation that both distract from one's meditative state—and the laughter that often accompanies the pose further aids the liberation from agitation! One is thereby able to return to a calm and alert meditative state.

As with all magical movement techniques, one completes the movement with the shaking, visualization, exhalation, and the vocalizations of *ha* and *phat* as described above.

The Benefits of the Principal Root Magical Movements

In reviewing the benefits of the first six root magical movements, Shardza's *Commentary* clusters the benefits of the first five root magical movements as a group, stating again that the first five root magical movements help overcome the five poisons or afflictions:

> As for the benefits of these five, as summarized from *Quintessential Oral Insructions*: "The door to the channel of the five poisons is closed, and the door to the channel of primordial wisdom is opened. The five aggregates are purified in their own place, and the *mandala* of the five enlightened bodies is perfected. The five elements are controlled and the five radiant lights arise."

Here we have the five correspondences that each magical movement is said to activate. The channel related to the poisons (the right one) closes down, and the one related to the primordial wisdoms (the left one) opens up. The five aggregates are the basic components to our psycho-physical organism: consciousness, form, formation, feeling, and conception. By purifying them one's organism becomes nothing less than a buddha. The five physical elements—space, earth, air, fire, and water—are the basic components of the physical realm. The "mandalas of the five enlightened bodies," or buddha dimensions, are the truth dimension, the complete or radiant dimension, the manifested dimension, the essential dimension, and the fully awakened dimension. People familiar with Buddhism may know the first three by their Sanskrit names of *dharmakaya*, *sambhogakaya*, and *nirmanakaya*; in Bön they go by the Tibetan names of *bonku*, *dzogku*, and *tulku*. Finally, according to Tibetan tradition, wisdom has five qualities, sometimes called five wisdoms, here referred to as "essential lights." These are emptiness, mirror-like, equanimity, discrimination, and all-accomplishing. Note how each magical movement correlates to five separate categories: one of the five elements, one of the five aggregates, one of the five poisons, one of the five wisdoms, and one of the five buddha dimensions (see chart 1 below). In addition to these five correspondences, the text speaks about five mandalas that arise with a successful practice: these are the purified chakras.

Before providing a detailed description of the benefit of each magical movement from the point of view of the five correspondences, *Quintessential Oral Instructions* instructs us to integrate the experiences of magical movement with our everyday activities, both day and night. That is to say, hold the taste of the effects of the practice in your mind as you go about your day, and while falling asleep and waking, in order to bring those insights into all that you do.

The Benefit of Striking the Athlete's Hammer to Overcome Anger

> The benefits of striking the athlete's hammer are that the path that is the space channel liberates, and the door to the anger channel closes. Having liberated the consciousness aggregate,

> the pure realm of the truth buddha dimension (*bonku*) dawns. The space essence dawns and the collection of the four diseases is liberated. Having liberated the object of knowledge in its own place, the external, internal, and secret interferences are cleared. Space does not set and the emptiness wisdom dawns.

The text claims that all four diseases (wind, bile, phlegm, and the combination of these three) will be liberated. The element of space is mastered, and the wisdom of emptiness arises. The truth dimension of the buddha is accessed. As the external, internal, and secret obstacles are cleared, the aggregate of consciousness can rest naturally in its own place, undisturbed. This is beautifully articulated in the last line: "Space does not set and emptiness wisdom dawns."

The Benefit of the Skylight of Primordial Wisdom to Overcome Delusion

> As for the benefits of the "skylight of primordial wisdom to overcome delusion," having liberated the form aggregate in its own place, the essence of earth dawns. The complete buddha dimension dawns, and the expanded mandalas are seen. The door to the mental fogginess channel closes and the mirror-like wisdom is completed. Form is mastered, and mountains and rocks are not obstructive.

By closing the door to the delusion channel, confusion, or mental cloudiness, is dispelled, the mirror-like wisdom is realized, and the practitioner is granted access to the complete buddha dimension (*dzogku*). Having mastery over the aggregate of form, the element of earth is also mastered, and mountains, rocks, or any other form cannot obstruct one's clarity. In other words, as the mind is as clear as a mirror, and none of the appearances disturb its clarity.

The Benefit of Rolling the Four Limbs Like Wheels to Overcome Pride

> As for the benefits of "rolling the four limbs like wheels to overcome pride," the formations aggregate liberates, and the air essence dawns. The essential buddha dimension is seen and the mandala of the three buddha dimensions dawn. The door to the pride channel closes and one realizes the wisdom of equanimity. One masters the air element, and the skill of swift walking is strengthened and expanded.

Here, the practitioner has access to the essential buddha dimension, opening to the mandala of the first three buddha dimensions (i.e., the truth, complete, and manifested dimensions). This brings about the closing of the door to the pride channel and allows the manifestation of the wisdom of equanimity. After mastering the air element, and liberating the aggregate of formations, one can achieve the special power of swift walking, described as being able to walk slightly above the ground and cover great distances quickly. In other words, by mastering the air element, one can move like air.

The Benefit of Loosening the Corner of the Braided Knot to Overcome Attachment

> As for the benefits of "loosening the corner of the braided knot to overcome attachment," the feeling aggregate is liberated and the fire essence dawns. The diverse manifested buddha dimensions (*tulku*) are completed and the manifestation mandala dawns. The door to the attachment channel closes and the discriminating wisdom dawns. One masters the fire element, and the fire and warmth of the yogic inner heat blazes.

Attachment here means that one is trapped by desire or lust. The loosening of the braided knot of attachment, I believe, is an effective metaphor. The power of the fire element liberates the aggregate of feeling and allows the practitioner to have access to the various manifested buddha dimensions and mandalas, which can be understood as the purified chakras. Therefore, the door to the desire channel closes, allowing discriminating wisdom to dawn, and with it, the possibility of understanding the uniqueness of each manifestation within their varieties is made possible. Here the magical movements are closely connected to the practice of yogic heat, or *tummo*: as one masters the fire element, the warmth that is developed through the yogic inner-heat practice seems to be maintained without much effort.

The Benefit of Waving the Silk Tassel Upward to Overcome Jealousy

> As for the benefits of "waving the silk tassel upward to overcome jealousy," the aggregate of conceptions is liberated and the essence of water dawns. The fully awakened buddha dimension is complete, and the five mandalas dawn. The door to the jealousy channel closes and the all-accomplishing wisdom expands. One masters the water element and has no lethargy.

When the element of water dawns, the aggregate of conceptions is liberated, allowing the practitioner to have access to the fully awakened buddha dimension and so the five mandalas dawn. Through closing the door to the jealousy channel, one is aware of the quality of the all-accomplishing wisdom. After mastering the water element, one overcomes lethargy, finding this relaxed, stable, water-like state of mind to be a support for understanding the harmonious existence of different phenomena as spontaneously perfected. This is very important: it is like a *purer* water-element quality, since water can also bring too much comfort and thus actually increase lethargy. However, the benefit here is that one masters that quality with balance; relaxed but not lethargic.

The Benefit of the Stance of a Tigress's Leap to Overcome Drowsiness and Agitation

> Regarding the "stance of a tigress's leap to overcome drowsiness and agitation," the force of the powerful wind is complete, and

Chart 1: Table of Correlations of Root Magical Movement Set

Magical movement	Element dawns / channel opens	Poison clears / channel closes	Aggregate liberated	Wisdom dawns / accomplishment	Buddha dimension dawns / seen
Striking the Athlete's Hammer	Space	Anger	Consciousness	Emptiness	Truth
Skylight of Primordial Wisdom	Earth	Delusion	Form	Mirror-like	Complete
Rolling the Four Limbs like Wheels	Air	Pride	Formations	Equanimity	Essential
Loosening the Corner of the Braided Knot	Fire	Attachment	Feeling	Discrimination	Manifested
Waving the Silk Tassel Upward	Water	Jealousy	Conceptions	All-Accomplishing	Truly/fully awakened

> lethargic mental fogginess purifies in its own place. The winds and the mind enter the central channel from below, and their moving liberates in its own place.

This sixth magical movement has no complex correspondences as do the first five. Instead, as those five are accomplished, and the elements and so forth balanced, one stays in that balance by releasing drowsiness and agitation. The entering of the winds and the mind into the central channel (as is also mentioned in the benefits of the foundational magical movement cycle) is a very important characteristic of higher tantric practices. Allowing obstacles to purify and liberate in their own place is an exemplary Dzogchen trait. As the obstacles are liberated, so are conceptual thoughts. Ponlob Thinley Nyima adds that the agent of the moving mind that liberates the accumulated thoughts into the central channel is also connected to two advanced practices of Dzogchen, "breakthrough" and "direct leap vision," or *trekcho* and *togal*. Because magical movement works with both the subtle body physiology and the mind resting in its own natural place, it is said that it conforms well with Dzogchen practice.

Root Magical Movement Set That Clears Away Obstacles

The root magical movement set that clears away obstacles is believed by tradition to have been designed by Togme Shigpo, a direct student of Pongyal Tsenpo. It first appears in *Quintessential Oral Instructions* as a set of five magical movements, to which Shardza, in his *Commentary*, adds a sixth. Drugyalwa did not include this in his presentation in the thirteenth century, so we can only conclude that it was a later addition, perhaps first added by Shardza himself or one of his teachers—perhaps in order to make a parallel to the six principal root magical movements.

The six root magical movements that clear away obstacles are:

1. Duck Drinking Water
2. Wild Yak Butting Sideways
3. Female Donkey Lying Down to Sleep

4. Kestrel Hovering in the Wind
5. Rolling Up the Limits of the Four Continents
6. Extending the Limits of the Four Continents

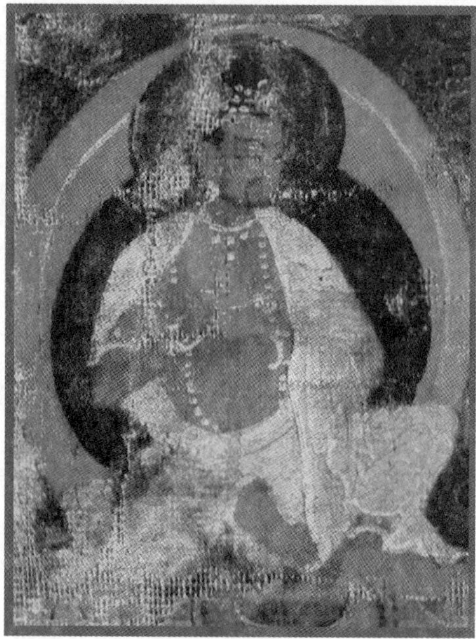

Togme Shigpo

Interestingly, *Quintessential Oral Instructions* teaches that the first five of these movements are performed while standing, but Shardza's sixth is done while sitting; in the root magical movement set it is the opposite—the first five are performed sitting and the sixth is done standing.

As with the root magical movements, these movements' names aid the practitioner in understanding the instruction. Note how the first four movements of this set have names of animals engaged in a particular action, which helps the practitioner to visualize the specific movement.

Duck Drinking Water

The first root magical movement that clears away obstacles is the "duck drinking water." In this particular posture, the practitioner is told to relate to the sense of being like a duck. Standing and straightening one's body, with both hands at the waist, thumbs pointing forward, one shifts the fronts of the feet open, heels close to each other and toes pointing outward diagonally, imitating a duck's stance. As one inhales and holds the breath in the neutral way, allowing the wind to spread pervasively, one first opens the chest area and then bends at the waist, stooping forward in a motion of reaching the head to the ground as if to drink water from it. Then, standing up, one slightly bends the head backward at the nape, keeping shoulders and chest open and relaxed, as though swallowing the water. One repeats the movement seven times, and concludes with the characteristic shaking of the limbs, while visualizing the stirring of all cyclic existence, exhaling the stale breath, and vocalizing *ha* and *phat*. One maintains the intention that all sentient beings are cleared from any obstacles. The opening of the chest relates to the space element, as we also saw in the first magical movement of the previous set, the "athlete's hammer to overcome anger." In the benefits section, we will see how the correlations continue and expand into those for overcoming physical illness.

Wild Yak Butting Sideways

In imitation of the sideways butting of a wild yak, the right leg is placed one step in front of the left, and, having inhaled and holding the wind in the neutral way, one places the weight of one's torso on the right leg. Then, following with the right shoulder and head, which creates the butting, one makes a little jump to place all the weight onto the left leg, which is now in front, and following with the left shoulder and head, which creates the butting to the left side, thus completing one movement. Perform this movement seven times, alternating the two sides, feeling the power of the butting without letting it disturb one's balance.

Although this movement looks very different than its parallel from the previous set, "skylight of wisdom," which is performed sitting and rolling back and forth, it has a similar function in terms of swirling internally to release mental fogginess and bring clarity to the mind of the practitioner. This clarity is heightened by the usual concluding movement of shaking the limbs, together with the exhalation of the stale breath, sounding *ha* and *phat,* and the prescribed visualization.

Female Donkey Lying Down to Sleep

"Female donkey lying down to sleep" is also performed while standing, with back straight and feet shoulder-width apart. With the hands at the waist, while stepping forward with the left leg, simultaneously one turns and twists with the torso downward to the left, with the right elbow trying to touch the left knee, as though one is a donkey who is turning her body halfway to lie on the ground to sleep. One then returns to full upright position and stepping with the right leg forward, bends and twists to the right, trying to reach the right knee with the left elbow. As one turns and brings the torso up slightly, it is like awakening from a sleeping posture. This is similar to the standing up on one's knees in "rolling the four limbs like a wheel," and here also one opens the chest and awakens the mind. "Female donkey lying down to sleep" follows a pattern of alternating between trying to go to sleep and rising seven times. It then concludes with the usual shaking of the limbs, together with the exhalation, visualization, and vocalizations.

Kestrel Hovering in the Wind

Ponlob Thinley Nyima explains that the kestrel is a small kind of hawk that is capable of holding its breath while hovering. In imitation of the bird, one stands with both feet together and both hands at the waist. One inhales and holds the breath in the neutral manner, maintaining a straight torso and allowing the pervasive wind to spread throughout the body. One then lifts the heels slightly, resting mostly on the balls of the feet. From that stance, one shifts the head toward the right side, following with the torso sideways and downward as far as one can go, subtly swaying the body like the hovering of the kestrel. One performs the same movement to the left and then returns to the center, looking skyward with a slight rising upward. After repeating the pattern right, left, and center seven times, one does the concluding shaking, exhalation, visualization, and vocalizations. The holding of the breath for all seven repetitions can be difficult in this movement. This in itself can bring more inner heat, activating the fire element. As in loosening the corner of the braided knot, the trap of attachment is liberated, especially at the end of the movement. In other words, after a long holding of the breath and guiding it with the kestrel-like movement throughout the whole torso, the exhalation releases obstacles, allowing one to connect to the clarity of the fire and the resting in the freed mind.

Rolling Up the Limits of the Four Continents

"Rolling up the limits of the four continents" is one of the movements that requires more coordination, as it involves crossing one leg across the thigh while standing and hopping, and while simultaneously crossing one's arms. Standing upright with feet shoulder-width apart, the arms resting by the sides and palms opened forward, one inhales and holds the breath in the neutral way. With a slight jump, one brings the right foot up above the left knee, touching the leg with the sole of the foot. Simultaneously, one crosses the arms over the chest, right over left, and places one's hands under the opposite armpits. The four continents are the four limbs, which are described as "rolling," as one alternates the legs and arms, jumping in this manner seven times to each side. The leg that crosses corresponds to the arm that is above when crossing. After alternating legs and arms seven times to each side, one concludes with the usual shaking, exhalation, visualization, and vocalizations.

Extending the Limits of the Four Continents

This final root magical movement that clears away obstacles is the one that Shardza added to the set. This movement may be difficult for most. Sitting in a cross-legged posture that is described here as "*vajra* cross-legged posture"—another name for the full lotus posture—one makes a fist with both hands with the thumbs inside, pressing on the base of the ring fingers, the gesture known as the *vajra* fist. Placing the top of the fists on the ground with palms facing inward, and loading one's weight on the fists, one raises one's body off the ground, rotating counterclockwise slightly before releasing. Each of the seven repetitions rotates the body further, until one has returned to the original position. In this way, one extends the limits of the four continents that are, again, the four limbs. While the fifth movement dispelled the obstacles by rotating the limbs, in this sixth movement the limbs are bound, and the full rotation of the whole body in that posture generates a sense of expansion that helps clear away obstacles. Upon conclusion one performs the usual concluding shaking, exhalation, visualization, and vocalizations.

The Benefits of the Root Magical Movement Set That Clears Away Obstacles

The *Commentary* describes the benefits of the root magical movement set that clears away obstacles as follows:

> The benefits of these, according to *Quintessential Oral Instructions*, are the following:
>
> The "duck" liberates from the diseases of the four consituents (phlegm, bile, wind, and the combination of the three) and opens the door of the channels of the space element; the "wild yak" liberates from the diseases of phlegm and opens the doors of the channels of the earth element; the "female donkey" liberates from diseases of bile and opens the doors of the channels of the air element; the "kestrel" liberates from diseases of heat and opens the doors of the channels of fire; and the "four continents" liberates from diseases of cold and opens the doors of the channels of water.

These benefits have interesting parallels with those of the previous set. Both sets follow the same order of the elements: space, earth, air, fire, and water, and the last movement of both is a combination of the five elements. The root set places more emphasis on the afflictive obstructions related to the mental obscurations, while the set of magical movements that clear away obstacles places more emphasis on diseases of the body. As for the collection of the four diseases mentioned in the benefits of the "duck drinking water," Ponlob Thinley Nyima explains that this refers to the imbalances of wind, of bile, of phlegm, and of the combination of the three. These are identical

Chart 2: Table of Correlations of Both Root Magical Movement Sets

Principal magical movement	Poison clears/ overcomes	Opening door of channel of element	Magical movement that clears away obstacles	Illness liberated
Striking the Athlete's Hammer	Anger	Space	**Duck Drinking Water**	Combination of four diseases
Skylight of Primordial Wisdom	Delusion	Earth	**Wild Yak Butting Sideways**	Diseases of phlegm
Rolling the Four Limbs like Wheels	Pride	Air	**Female Donkey Lying Down to Sleep**	Diseases of bile
Loosening the Corner of the Braided Knot	Attachment	Fire	**Kestrel Hovering in the Wind**	Diseases of heat
Waving the Silk Tassel Upward	Jealousy	Water	**Rolling the Four Continents**	Diseases of cold

to, and probably derive from, Tibetan medicine. In chart 2, the movements of both sets are shown side by side, to bring more clarity to the correlations between the two.

As for the common benefits of this set, the practice of these movements is said to "cause one to possess the power of speed-walking, to blaze the warmth of the body, and to reverse the aging process."

In brief, the root magical movement set, designed by Pongyal Tsenpo, is said to work by opening the door of the five elements and closing the door of the five poisons in order to allow primordial wisdom and its manifestation as the five buddha dimensions and the five lights to manifest. The root magical movement set that clears away obstacles, designed by Togme Shigpo, helps overcome illnesses so that the practitioner can actually have the experiences of mandalas and lights that arise from accessing one's primordial wisdom. These movements can also bring extraordinary powers through the manipulation of the winds, the focus of the mind and the body movements guiding them, such as speed-walking, reverse aging, and so forth. Simply stated, these root magical movements can bring mystical, medical, and magical results.

Branch Magical Movement Cycle

Similar to the root cycle, the branch magical movement cycle is composed of two sets: the main branches and the ancillary branches that clear away obstacles. Each set has five magical movements. Both are credited by the tradition to Lhundrub Muthur.

The five main branch magical movements are:

1. Natural Descent of the Four Elements
2. Peacock Drinking Water
3. Collecting the Four Stalks
4. Rolling the Four Upper and Lower Limbs
5. Striking the Four Braided Knots

This first set is practiced in order to gain outer and inner strength, while the second set is designed to clear away obstacles.

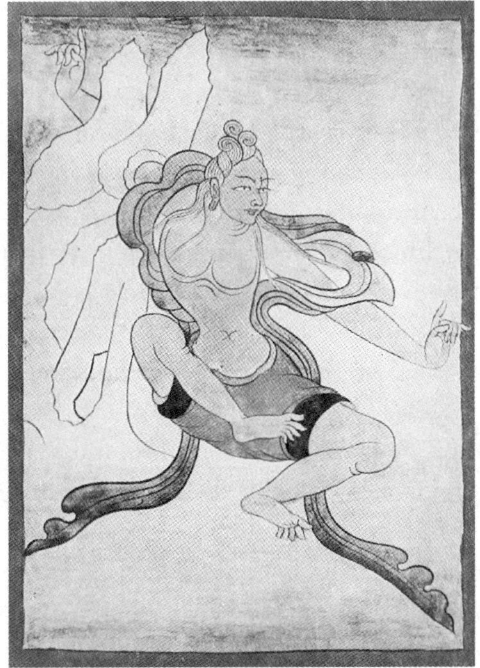

Lhundrub Muthur

Natural Descent of the Four Elements

In the first magical movement of this set, one assumes the cross-legged position and places the palms, pressing lightly, upon both thighs. As the forearms and torso are straightened, the channels are straightened too. Bringing the head and upper body down and forward with a slight shake toward the ground, one visualizes the motion as a smooth descent of the elements, like snowflakes falling to the ground. Coming back to an upright position, one is instructed to harmoniously move the head and torso down as before for a total of seven times. As this smooth descent and ascent is done, as in all movements, by holding the breath pervasively the inner obstacles dissolve smoothly too. With a sense of lightness at the end of the seven repetitions, one concludes with the standard shaking of the limbs along with the exhalation, visualization, and vocalizations.

Peacock Drinking Water

Seated with legs extended in front and parallel to each other, one crosses one's forearms behind one's back—having hands touching at thumbs and index fingers is also acceptable—with the thumbs pressing the ring fingers of each hand, the other fingers extended. Bending the body forward, one imagines going to drink water on the ground in front of oneself, with the forehead reaching toward the space in between the knees. As one raises the head again, twist it gently to the right over the shoulder, and then twist the head over the left shoulder. This is explained as the peacock checking to see who is around her. One then brings the head to the center, looks upward, and imagines finally swallowing the water. This entire sequence is repeated seven times. The movement stretches the channels so that the winds flow unruffled. The name is not just a way to describe the movement; taking its peacock allegory a step further, one can feel that one swallows the poisons and converts them into nurturing nectar or medicine. After feeling restored by the winds in that way, one concludes as usual.

Collecting the Four Stalks

The "four stalks," like the "four continents" in the previous set, refer here to the four limbs of the body. One takes a seated posture, with legs bent at the knees, the soles of the feet together. Grabbing the big toes with both hands one rocks backward and forward. While leaning backward, with the backbone on the ground, one stretches the arms and legs skyward, releasing the toes and allowing the limbs to separate, radiating outward in four directions. Rolling forward, one collects the four limbs like stalks and returns to the starting posture. After the openness from radiating the limbs, it can feel like retrieving nurturing qualities that are collected and gathered as one moves forward. Repeating this movement seven times with a sense of fulfillment, one concludes with the usual shaking of the limbs, exhalation, visualization, and vocalizations.

Rolling the Four Upper and Lower Limbs

Maintaining the seated posture, now in a full lotus position, this magical movement works with the limbs bound, rather than radiating and being brought together as in the previous magical movement. Grabbing the toes of each foot with one's fingers, one rolls backward, reaching with one's knees toward the ground. Then, rolling forward, with the knees touching the ground, still in lotus position, one brings the forehead forward and down, as far as one can reach—placing the forehead on the ground if possible. This back and forth movement can feel like the charging of a dynamo. Charging in that way seven times, one concludes as usual, with a strong sense of liberation in the exhalation, shaking, visualization, and vocalizations.

Striking the Four Braided Knots

The last magical movement of this set begins in the same full lotus posture as above and in the "extending the limits" movement from the previous set. However, in this movement one brings the right and left hands in between the cove of the knees, right hand to right leg, left hand to left leg, holding each calf from underneath. Inhaling and making sure that the neutral holding is settled, one hops up and and rotates the whole body counterclockwise, repeating seven times and returning to the initial position. His Holiness, the late Lungtok Tenpai Nyima, the former head of the Bön tradition, commented on the rotation of the pose, asserting that not only for this movement, but in general, when a Bön text does not indicate the direction, the rotation should always be in the "Bön way," i.e., counterclockwise (Buddhists, by contrast, mostly rotate clockwise).

As for the "four braided knots," I believe this refers to the limbs, and, actually, the "four-fold braided knot" might be a better way of conceiving it. The "striking," which here means hitting the ground each time—what Tibetans call *bep*—helps to release the knots, which again refer to an obstacle or a limitation. In other words, the knot is something that prevents the proper flow of the wind; the rotating and the *bep* unties the knots, allowing the winds to purify one's organism internally. Shardza's *Commentary* reaffirms that at the end of this set one must "shudder and shake the four limbs and recite the sounds *ha* and *phat*, as required in all magical movements."

Benefits of the Branch Magical Movement Cycle

Shardza's *Commentary* cites *Quintessential Oral Instructions* to lay out the benefits of these magical movements:

> One liberates from diseases of the four elements. Wind and mind penetrate the vital points making the body function well. Appearances are liberated as illusions, and attachment to deluded appearances is reversed. The strength of the body is increased. You obtain natural mastery over the four elements. External and internal obstacles are cleared, and the winds penetrate the vital points of the channels making the body function well. The oily blazing warmth of the body blazes radiantly. The excellent strength of the body is increased.

Similar to the root magical movements, especially the root magical movements that clear away obstacles, the elements correlate to illnesses in this set. Note that again when four elements are mentioned, they are omitting space, since it is the one that allow all the other four elements to exist. Both *Quintessential Oral Instructions* and the *Commentary* only mention general benefits of this set and do not enumerate separate benefits for each magical movement. However, we find here the addition of the obstacles related to the mind. Twice the passage translated above uses a Tibetan phrase that literally means "penetrate the vital points," which, as Ponlob Thrinley Nyima observes, is a well-known expression meaning that things are "functioning well." He explains it as being analogous to the gears of a machine being greased. The mention of the increase of the body oil, heat, and luminosity can be regarded as signs that the machine is in optimal performance mode and that the practitioner has conquered the elements—in particular, here, fire.

The Branch Magical Movement Set That Clears Away Obstacles

The branch magical movement set that clears away obstacles is also composed of five magical movements:

1. Great Garuda Flapping Its Wings
2. Peacock Shaking Off Water
3. Collecting the Four Limbs and Clearing Away Limitations
4. Antelope Galloping Sideways
5. Deer Shaking Sideways

Great Garuda Flapping Its Wings

The first of this set begins in a standing posture, ready to "fly." Standing upright like a vertical brush stroke, one extends the right arm skyward, the left arm along one's side. With a small jump, one bends the right arm to touch the right shoulder-blade with the hand, and simultaneously bends the right leg and touches the buttocks with the back of the right heel. *Quintessential Oral Instructions* explains that one should extend and contract the arm and leg simultaneously. One then performs the same movement on the left side. Alternating this movement with the right and left side seven times, one amply opens the chest area with each extension of the arm, or "wing," and feels lighter with the jumping, i.e., the "flying." The conclusion is as usual, shaking the limbs, exhaling sounding *ha* and *phat*, and visualizing the clearing away of obstacles from all beings, including oneself.

Peacock Shaking Off Water

Continuing in the standing posture, one extends one's arms in front of one's chest and brings them down to the ground around the feet. Shaking both hands simultaneously to the front, right, and left sides, one imagines shaking off water. The movement concludes by returning to the upright posture, and repeats seven times. The stretching and elongation of the arms helps in creating more internal space for the air to move. The shaking off of the water also creates a rippling effect in stirring oneself internally. This movement, as well as the antelope and the deer movements below, stretches the ability to hold one's breath—supported by the neutral holding and pervasive wind—and may be designed in part to increase the capacity to do so. One ends with the usual shaking, exhalation, and visualization, clearing away all that was shaken off.

Collecting the Four Limbs and Clearing Away Limitations

This difficult magical movement is the only one within this set that does not begin in a standing posture. Squatting down to rest on the sides of one's feet, without bending the back, with the knees spread out to the sides and the buttocks raised—if needed they can touch the ground—one collects the four limbs by touching the soles of the feet together and holding them with the hands. Hopping seven times forward and seven backward while maintaining this binding posture, one clears away limitations. These limitations can certainly be physical, such as flexibility and strength, but also energetic and mental. In that regard, it can relate to overcoming the collection of the four diseases as part of the physical limitations and to clearing away one's conceptual mind as part of the mental limitations. One concludes as usual.

Antelope Galloping Sideways

This long magical movement has twenty-eight steps. Standing on the right foot while holding the ankle and upper part of the left foot with the left hand, one places the sole of that foot in the bottom-right side of the intestines. In this posture, one hops forward on the right leg while simultaneously shaking the right hand toward the right hip. Taking seven small hops forward, one then turns around and takes seven small hops in the other direction. Still holding the breath, one changes the positions of the legs, standing on the left leg and holding the right foot with the right hand and placing it on the bottom-left side of the intestines. Again one hops, now on the left leg, seven times forward, and turning around, hops seven times backward. This movement creates some internal stirring, which, together with the release provoked with the shaking of the hands toward the hips, helps to clear away obstacles. After twenty-eight steps, one is ready to exhale thoroughly, releasing external, internal, and secret obstacles. One concludes with the usual shaking, exhalation, visualization, and vocalizations.

Deer Shaking Sideways

Similar in some ways to the preceding movement, the "deer shaking sideways" pushes the limits of the holding of one's breath. Standing upright with the arms at the side, the sole of the right foot presses perpendicularly against the side of the left calf, forming the shape of a skylight or triangular window. In that posture, one extends the arms behind one's back with the hands crossing in the same position as the "peacock drinking water"—crossing one's forearms behind one's back, with the thumbs pressing the ring fingers of each hand and the other fingers extended. It is also acceptable to not cross the arms, as long as the fingers are touching properly, as before. One makes a small hop forward and, with each hop, bends the torso, shoulders, and head forward and then back up vertically three times, while simultaneously making a downward movement with the hands. After hopping forward seven times, with three bows each time, one turns around and does seven hops with three bows each with the left leg now raised against the right leg. Shardza emphasizes that the whole movement is done "with one inhalation." And as we know, all these magical movements are done with one inhalation, but he may be emphasizing how this one stretches our breath-holding capacity. This extensive movement concludes with shaking, a well-deserved exhalation, vocalization, and visualization.

Benefits of the Branch Magical Movement Set That Clears Away Obstacles

In his *Commentary* Shardza states:

> The obstacles from the elements are liberated. The doors to the

> channel of the elements are opened. The elements are balanced. You are unharmed by the collection of the four diseases.

Interestingly, the passage in *Quintessential Oral Instructions* that Shardza is here claiming to quote actually gives five elements instead of four, while it continues to state that "the door of the channel of the four elements is opened." Again, the variation most likely is a matter of whether or not the element of space is included; it is sometimes considered as the container of the four elements and not an element in itself. In any event, as the obstacles from the elements are liberated and the door of the element's channel is opened, the elements come into balance, and thus one cannot be harmed by disease. This is in accordance with the Tibetan medical theory, which states that illness is the result of an imbalance of one's elements. In magical movement, the restoration to balance is done by the pneumatic force of the winds guided by the physical movements and the focus of one's mind.

Distinctive Magical Movement Set That Clears Away Specific Obstacles

There are two sets that are named "distinctive": the distinctive magical movement set that clears away specific obstacles, and the distinctive magical movement set that clears away common obstacles. The first set is composed of five movements that each clear away the obstacles that are specific of the head, torso, arms, lower body (specifically the stomach), and legs, respectively. The second set focuses on clearing away obstacles that are in common for the whole body.

The first, the distinctive magical movement set that clears away specific obstacles, resembles the foundational set in its clearing away or purifying of obstacles from the different parts of the body. One might think of it as the "distinctive foundational set," since both have five movements relating to different parts of the body. One important difference between them is that in the foundational set the clearing is done through a massage or sweeping of the winds with one's hands in the different areas of one's body, while in the distinctive set the clearing of obstacles is mostly internal and the winds guided by the movement of that particular area of the body. They are:

1. Rotating and Nodding the Head
2. Swinging the Binding Chains of the Torso
3. Grasping like the Raven's Claws
4. *Vajra* Self-Rotation of the Stomach
5. Camel's Fighting Stance

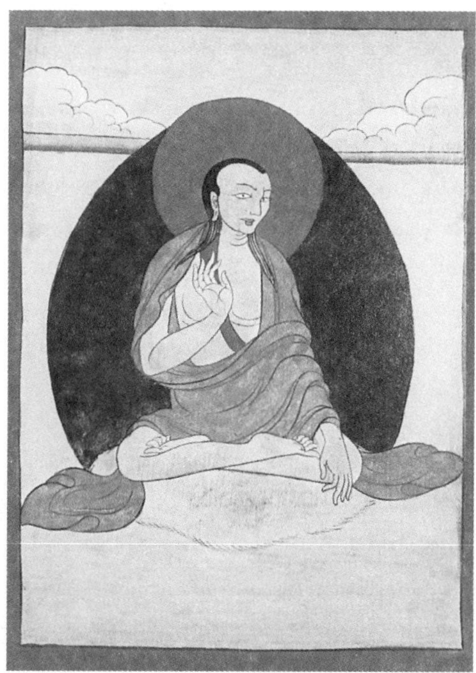

Orgom Kundul

Rotating and Nodding the Head

The first magical movement of this set starts with the gradual clearing of the body, beginning with the head. Sitting in the cross-legged posture, one places both hands on top of the thighs—or at the inguinal crease—which helps straighten the back along with the inner channels. Holding the breath in the usual neutral manner, one rotates the head seven times counterclockwise and seven times clockwise, which one is advised to do so slowly. The movement guides the pervasive wind in order to help clear away obstacles of the head as one imagines the wind internally spiraling up and "waking up" all the sense organs in the head. Still holding the breath, one continues with a front–back movement of the head, which is also repeated seven times and produces a similar awakening sensation. The conclusion is the usual visualization together with the shaking of the limbs and the exhalation with *ha* and *phat*.

Swinging the Binding Chains of the Torso

The next pose is done in a kneeling position. With one's knees planted on the ground and the legs crossed behind at the ankles, one places most of one's weight forward. One's arms cross around the straightened torso, holding the opposite shoulders. One twists this "chained" torso by first bringing the right shoulder toward the left knee and rotating counterclockwise seven times, then bringing the left shoulder to the right knee, rotating clockwise seven times. The constrained torso feels liberated internally; the movement helps the opening and clearing of the obstacles in the torso. The conclusion here is as usual.

Grasping like the Raven's Claws

This movement, which has been described as looking like ravens fighting, is performed while sitting in the "bodhisattva posture"—sometimes also called "royal posture" or "half lotus." The left leg is flat against the ground with the foot tucked into the groin; the right leg is bent with the foot placed slightly in front of the body. This pose will be repeated in several other magical movements below. One places one's arms on each side of the body with the hands clinched loosely like claws, the thumb pressing the tips of the other fingers, the fingers pointing outward away from the body. Raising and extending first the right arm, the palm and fingers extend out to that side and return back to the starting position. One then performs the movement with the left arm. Alternating between the right and left arms, one repeats the movement seven times on each side. One imagines the clearing away of obstacles from the arms. The conclusion of the movement is with the usual visualization, shaking, exhalation, and vocalizations.

Vajra *Self-Rotation of the Stomach*

Although the texts instruct one to sit in the bodhisattva posture, for those who can, the lotus position is preferable in this pose in order to keep the torso and channels straight. Crossing the right and left arms by holding the opposite elbow, one embraces the outer ribcage and stomach. It is also acceptable to cross the arms at the stomach and hold one's sides. Then, one rotates at the waist and stomach seven times, first counterclockwise and then seven times clockwise. This movement can be said to release subtle obstacles from the navel energetic center, which is the hub of the area. One concludes as with all other magical movements.

Camel's Fighting Stance

The last magical movement of this set is focused on the legs, but it engages the whole body. Sitting on the floor, one extends the forearms between the legs, and reaches under the calves to hold the big toes with the hands. Rolling backward, planting the nape of the neck on the ground, one extend the legs and arms vertically like brush strokes, stirring and shaking in the air, as if fighting. "Having done that," *Quintessential Oral Instructions* states, "complete the turning," which is to say, return to the bound position. The opening and contracting of the body and limbs in these movements guides the winds to spread and contract through the channels, clearing away obstacles of the whole body. The external movement reflects well the inner mandala-dynamism. As with most magical movements, here too one repeats the movement seven times. One is instructed to conclude as usual with the shaking the four limbs and the vocalization of *ha* and *phat* and so forth.

Benefits of the Distinctive Magical Movement Set That Clears Away Specific Obstacles

In his *Commentary* Shardza describes the benefits of the distinctive magical movement set that clears away individual obstacles:

> As for the benefits, the perspective of Orgom Kundul is that all the cooperative conditions of heat, cold, wind, bile, and demons are cleared. Also, the diseases of each of the limbs are cleared.

For the first time we find among the benefits a direct mention of clearing away the demonic forces that are believed by Tibetans to cause illness and otherwise obstruct well-being. However the modern practitioner understands this—literally, as malicious beings in the world, as energies, or as metaphors for observable phenomena—the magical movements promise a means to surmount them.

Distinctive Magical Movement Set That Clears Away Common Obstacles

The second set of the distinctive magical movement cycle is the last magical movement set. It contains five magical movements; however, since one of them is subdivided into three parts, it actually becomes seven magical movements. Also, as we'll see, some of these movements were designed by Yangton Chenpo and others by his son, Bumje Ö. In contrast to its preceding set, which focused on specific parts of the body, these movements clear away common obstacles from the whole mind-energy-body system. They are:

1. Shaking the Depths of the Ocean
2. Loosening the Nine Braided Knots
3. Disciplining and Loosening the Channels
4. Chinese Woman Weaving Silk, Part One
5. Chinese Woman Weaving Silk, Part Two
6. Chinese Woman Weaving Silk, Part Three
7. Bouncing Jewel

Shaking the Depths of the Ocean

For the first of this set one sits in the bodhisattva posture and holds the legs under the calves with both hands. Hopping to raise the whole body with strength gathered internally, one rotates seven times counterclockwise and

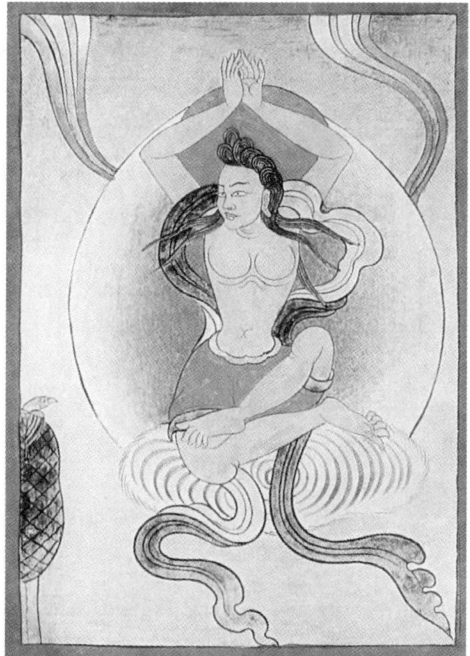

Yangton Chenpo

then seven times clockwise. This movement bears the name of the visualization that the yogin or practitioner creates in every magical movement, the shaking of the oceanic depths of cyclic existence. Thus, this movement emphasizes the shaking and then clearing of one's own obstacles together with those of all sentient beings. One should conclude as usual, with visualization, shaking, exhalation, and vocalization, and the sense of relief and joy.

Loosening the Nine Braided Knots

The "nine braided knots" that are loosened, or liberated, refer to the nine parts of the movement. Sitting with the soles of the feet on the ground and the knees bent, legs half-extended, one taps the body with both palms seven times in each of six places: the crown of the head, the forehead, the nape of the neck, the top of the right and left shoulders, the right and left hip bone, and above the right and left knees. One follows by tapping the ground with the feet, with an emphasis on the heels. Then, planting the palms of both hands on the ground alongside the body, one elevates the body to the sky three times. Some teachers add the instruction here to kick like a horse at this point and then bring the legs back down with the soles of the feet on the ground. Finally, still holding the breath, one stands up and jumps upward, returning to sit in the lotus posture, repeating this three times. This last motion is called "the great descent from stars to earth." The six taps with the hands, the tapping with the feet, the standing on the hands, and the great descents make nine parts of this magical movement, freeing all the areas involved. One concludes in a standing posture with the usual visualization, shaking, exhalation, and vocalization. This is quite a strenuous movement, probably the hardest of all, both in terms of holding the air for such a long time and the challenge of the physical posture.

Disciplining and Loosening the Channels

This magical movement is the only one in the text that has its own distinct visualization. Standing with legs together and the hands holding the waist with thumbs forward and four fingers back, one visualizes the three channels and six energetic centers or chakras, with a Tibetan syllable at each center:

- At the principal wheel of the crown an *A* ཨ
- At the throat an *Om* ཨོཾ
- At the heart center a *Hung* ཧཱུྃ
- At the wheel of the soles of the feet a *Yam* ཡཾ
- At the perineum (secret energy center) a *Ram* རཾ
- At the navel a *Kham* ཁཾ

Through the visualization and holding of the breath, one heats up the channels and the whole body-energy-mind system with the fire of inner heat. One visualizes that the *Ram* at the secret chakra ignites with fire, which heats up the channels and reaches the three main syllables *A*, *Om*, and *Hung*, at crown, throat, and heart chakras. These melt into light, transforming into three "drops" or *thiklés* (pronounced something like "tik-lay") of white, red, and azure colors, respectively. The three *thiklés* then dissolve, flowing down into the green *Yam* syllables, one at each of the soles of the feet. That activates both *Yam* syllables, spreading the winds which flow up through the legs and into the perineum area, blazing there in the fire of the red *Ram* syllable. Rising next to the yellow/gold *Kham* syllable at the navel chakra, the fire melts the *Kham* into nectar, which then falls down like drops. The fire of the *Ram* syllable is thusly enhanced by the nectar drops, and through the power of one's visualization, it rises as wind, fire, and golden light that clear away all the karmic latencies, predispositions, and obstacles of the three times (past, present, and future). With that visualization and neutral holding, one jumps in one's place, striking the buttocks with the heels at each of the seven jumps. The text describes it as being like a gallop. With each jump, the fire increases, fueled by the pervasive wind. One turns around and performs seven more galloping jumps. One imagines that it transforms into a powerful light that clears away obstacles as it spreads, clearing and burning external, internal, and secret obstacles. The spreading of the light upward, externally helped by the heel kicks, causes the light and wind to pervade like sun rays throughout the whole body, in the mandalic way described before.

Benefits of the First Three Movements of the Distinctive Magical Movement Set That Clears Away Common Obstacles

Both *Quintessential Oral Instructions* and Shardza's *Commentary* pause here to describe the benefits of the first three movements. Shardza begins with crediting the first three magical movements of this set to Yangton Chenpo, who is said to have taught them to his son Bumje Ö:

> One is liberated from all outer and inner obstacles: the cooperative conditions of the elements and all kinds of diseases. All defects of the channels, winds, and drops are cleared. The five winds penetrate the vital points. One obtains mastery of speed-walking, the blazing of blissful warmth, and the four elements. The motion of the hordes of thoughts naturally clears, and nonconceptual experiences of bliss and clarity arise. An experience of nonconceptual bliss and clarity arises.

The reference to "all kinds of disease" means the collection of four diseases (wind, bile, phlegm, and the combination of all three) as we have seen earlier. If we think of all kinds of disease from the Tibetan medical perspective, there would be three additional combinations: wind-bile, bile-phlegm, and wind-phlegm, making a total of seven. These could be the causes, which, together with the cooperative conditions due to the elements not being in balance, can bring disharmony or unbalance to one's mind-energy-body system. Therefore, these three magical movements can liberate the practitioner from such humor imbalance, as well as from external, internal, and secret obstacles.

In other words, through the performance of these magical movements, any flaw in the energetic body constituted by channels, winds, and *thiklés* is cleared away or dispelled by the inner mandala-dynamic power, bringing an overall balance. The five winds then penetrate and open the five chakras. As they open, they allow the flow of the winds, positively affecting the mind. The marvelous powers mentioned are the signs of success, not the goals. From the Bön and Buddhist perspective the most important result of the practice is the dissolution of thoughts, which provides the ability to abide in one's natural mind in experiences of bliss and clarity.

The five winds that flow through the wheels or chakras are the same ones as in Tibetan medicine, mentioned in the introduction, and correspond to the five elements. The *Mother Tantra*, a text from which Shardza quotes extensively, clearly renders the correspondences between the five winds, the five channel-and-wind (*tsalung*) movements and the same five elements which we have already seen above. Following that source: the upward-moving wind is related to the earth element and flows through the throat and crown chakras; the life-force wind is related to the space element and flows through the heart chakra; the fire-like wind is related to the fire element and flows through the navel chakra; the pervasive wind is usually related to the whole central channel (that starts at chakra of the union of the channels), and the downward-clearing wind is related to the water element and flows through the secret chakra. These correlations reaffirm that these magical movements are not only part of a spiritual endeavor but are also methods of healing that are closely linked with the Tibetan medical system.

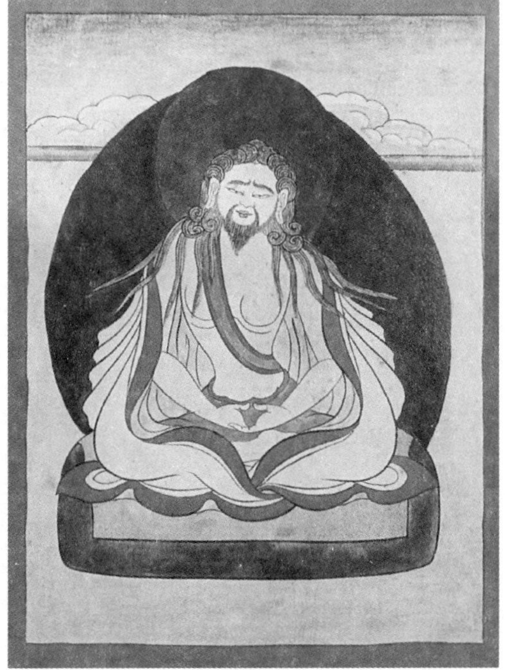

Bumje Ö

Chinese Woman Weaving Silk, Part One

The next three magical movements of this set are called "Chinese woman weaving silk," which is in three parts. Although each is a distinct magical movement, they are, as indicated by their name, closely related. In fact, both *Quintessential Oral Instructions* and *Experiential Transmission* consider them to be three stages of one movement. It is worth noting that this is the only movement with a name involving a human being—up to now we have only had metaphors involving animal behaviors. The woman weaving the silk is Chinese simply because Tibetans obtained their silk from China, and she is a woman because men rarely wove silk.

The first movement begins with taking a stance that evokes both the weaver and her loom. The loom is created first with right leg bent with the right knee up and the right hand holding the ankle. The left leg is lifted by the left arm, by reaching under the leg and holding the toes. In that position one moves one's left leg in seven circular motions, first inwardly and then outwardly, which simulates the weaving. This is then repeated with the other side. *Quintessential Oral Instructions* concludes this magical movement with a specific instruction to straighten the legs and the arms and to exhale, clearing all stale air, with the usual shaking, visualizations, and vocalizations.

Chinese Woman Weaving Silk, Part Two

Lying down on the right side, like the Buddha at the moment of his death, one closes the right nostril with the forefinger of the right hand and brings the thumb to carefully press the carotid artery. With the left hand, one grabs the left foot and performs seven circular "weaving" motions outward and seven inward. *Quintessential Oral Instructions* only mentions the inward rotation, possibly simply assuming the outward, while *Experiential Transmission* includes both explicitly and so does the *Commentary*. Still holding the breath, lying now on the left side, one repeats the seven outward circular "weaving" motions and seven inward . Then, standing or sitting, one performs the usual concluding shaking, visualization, exhalation, and vocalizations. This second part of the "Chinese woman weaving silk" is also said to be an important secondary practice for enhancing the "direct leap vision" practice (*togal*).

Chinese Woman Weaving Silk, Part Three

Sitting with one's legs bent, the knees pointing outward, one balances backward with the arms slightly lifted, holding the legs by the big toes—one can also hold the ankles instead. Alternating the legs, one brings each foot inward to touch the heel to the inside of the hipbone, or sit bone, almost touching the secret chakra in the perineum/genital area. One repeats this movement alternating seven times with each leg. *Quintessential Oral Instructions* and *Experiential Transmission* both describe this process as "the legs stretch, bend, alternating." The conclusion is with the usual shaking, exhalation, and visualization.

Benefits of Chinese Woman Weaving Silk

As with the first three movements of this set, the texts pause here to consider the benefits of "Chinese woman weaving silk" before proceeding to the last movement. According to Shardza's *Commentary*, citing *Quintessential Oral Instructions,*

> The first part of the "Chinese woman weaving silk" magical movement opens the door of the left channel, and wisdom increases. The female wind penetrates the vital points and pacifies agitation and the proliferation of thoughts.
>
> The second closes the door of the right channel and cuts off the continuous flow of mental afflictions. Mastery over the coarse winds is obtained and torpor and dullness are dispelled.
>
> The third opens the door of the central channel and trains the neutral wind. Mastery of appearances and mind is obtained and nonconceptual primordial wisdom arises.

The benefits of the "Chinese woman weaving silk" are thus considerable. The first movement opens the left—the female, or wisdom—channel, the second closes the right—the male, or affliction—channel, and the third one opens the central channel. More plainly stated, the first movement opens the wisdom channel, bringing in the female wind and pacifying discursive thoughts. Then, in the second, by closing the affliction channel and conquering the coarse wind, torpor and dullness are liberated. And finally, by mastering the neutral wind in the central channel, one is no longer distracted by appearances and mental "tricks" and thus nonconceptual primordial wisdom dawns.

The opening of the left channel in the first part of this magical movement with the wind is expressed slightly differently, according to our three source texts. While the *Commentary* mentions the female wind as penetrating the vital points, or, as we mentioned earlier, making the energetic system run well, *Quintessential Oral Instructions* mentions it as a distilled wind that penetrates the essential points. In *Experiential Transmission*, it is the coarse wind that penetrates the essential points

For the second part, all three texts are in agreement regarding the benefits: the closing of the door of the right channel and thus the cutting off of the continuity of the path of afflictions. All three also agree that one obtains natural power over the coarse wind, purifying torpor and dullness. *Experiential Transmission* mentions the coarse wind in both the first and second parts within the benefits, but I believe this is an error in the text, either of the author or of later copyists. Following the other texts, it would seem more sensible to have the first one be the gentle wind, the second one the coarse wind, and the third one the neutral wind.

There is also some slight variation regarding the third part of the magical movement. *Quintessential Oral Instructions* and *Experiential Transmission* both read "the two winds pierce the essential points and one obtains natural power over the external and internal." I believe that here the external and internal refer to the obstacles. *Quintessential Oral Instructions* concludes this part by stating: "the general flows are even," while *Experiential Transmission* refers to all three parts of the "Chinese woman weaving silk" magical movement, stating that they "teach the general flows." Neither mention the opening of the central channel here as Shardza's *Commentary* does in the passage translated above. The central channel is known for uniting and, in doing so, making the flow of the wind even, so it is possible to presume that both earlier texts assumed the opening of the central channel, and that Shardza makes it explicit.

We can also understand the benefits of the three together by thinking that all three parts of the "Chinese woman weaving silk" magical movement instruct the practitioner in the flow of the winds, left, right, and center. In that way, one is able to balance them and especially master the neutral wind, the most important for performing the magical movement. At the same time, one can control one's mind and have power over appearances and perceptions.

Bouncing Jewel

This is the thirty-ninth magical movement and the last one of our text. Sitting in the bodhisattva posture, one brings the arms parallel in front and forms the "jewel" by clasping the hands together with interlaced fingers, leaving the two forefingers pointing forward, almost like a gun, and the left thumb pressing on the top of the right thumb. Contracting the arms, one brings that jewel toward oneself hitting all areas of the chest with the jewel, while simultaneously vocalizing *phat* with each hit. After hitting as many times as possible, which is accompanied with deep inner stirring, one shakes and exhales with *ha* and *phat* as usual.

Quintessential Oral Instructions and *Experiential Transmission* both assert that the movement "clears the obstacles of the treasure of the torso." The Tibetan term used to instruct the striking of the chest and can be rendered poetically as "inspiring the heart."

Benefits of Bouncing Jewel

While both *Quintessential Oral Instructions* and *Experiential Transmission* describe the benefit of this magical movement, Shardza oddly overlooks it in his *Commentary*. *Quintessential Oral Instructions* explains:

> The benefits are: maintaining the heart wind in the chest treasure and liberating from the impure diseases.

Ponlob Thinley Nyima explains that in this movement the pressure brought by the breath in the torso is removed, like a "pressure cooker," with each *phat* vocalization and thumping, concluding with the total relief of the area. In this way, this movement is said to be particularly beneficial for heart problems. It seems that the more one is able to maintain the wind in the central channel and the heart as its center, the more physical and mental diseases are liberated. This would be something truly appealing to undertake as a research study within a modern Western medical framework.

Although in his *Commentary* Shardza does not describe the benefits for this magical movement, he does add a recommendation that would seem to apply to all magical movements, placed as it is as the concluding advice for the entire sequence of magical movements:

> Thus, in conclusion, rest easefully for a moment in a meditative equipoise, a state that is effortless, naturally liberated, free of action, and beyond the intellect.

In other words, through the practice of these magical movements, one can effortlessly clear or liberate one's illnesses, afflictions, and subtle mental disturbances, and thus abide uncontrived in the state of mind beyond intellect. One enters and is able to rest in meditative equipoise in one's own natural state of mind. And as the lamas advise us, rest with full awareness at the end of each session of magical movement practice.

There is nothing else that I can add here, except to reiterate how crucial this point is in understanding the impact that performing these magical movements can have on the experience of the practitioner. So, as Shardza concludes in his colophon, "may they become the conditions for giving birth to extraordinary experiences and realizations."

CHAPTER THREE

Making Magic Together

Historical Context: The Bön Religion

TIBETAN RELIGIOUS TRADITIONS are rich in mind-body practices used for spiritual development in the quest for enlightenment, and some, like magical movement, also used for physical, emotional, and mental well-being.

Magical movement is a distinctive Tibetan practice of physical yoga in which breath and concentration of the mind are integrated as crucial components in conjunction with particular body movements, like the ones we saw in the last chapter. These magical movements are part of the Bön Zhang Zhung Aural Transmission lineage. This is a very important Dzogchen lineage in Bön, as it has been uninterruptedly transmitted from teacher to disciple. These teachings were first transmitted mind-to-mind (from teacher to disciple), then through signs, then orally (from where it takes its name), and, finally, written. However, the fact that it is now written does not entail that the other kinds of transmission are not active. That is also part of the magic!

It may also be important to note here why we are calling it *aural* transmission. After being transmitted mind-to-mind, and then through symbols, it was transmitted through a bamboo cane from the mouth of a teacher to the ear of the disciple/student in order to make sure nothing was lost. It also prevented the teachings from being heard by those who were not ready for them. The act of hearing well as one receives this transmission is *nyen* in Tibetan, which is translated as *aural*—thus *aural* transmission. The spoken aspect of the teacher's instructions is *zhal shes* in Tibetan, and these terms are the structure of the teachings in the written text—maybe the invisible bamboo cane, as you read the translation of the *Commentary* in appendix 1.

Zhang Zhung is an area west of Tibet, and a cradle of much of the Bön tradition. And despite some claims in favor of roots in Indian esoteric Buddhism, a full and accurate history of magical movements is yet to be written. Contemporary Tibetan religious leaders and scholars date magical movement practices back to at least the eighth century. In fact, they claim that different kinds of magical movements, such as those of this book, were practiced much earlier than that and preserved only as an oral tradition. Certainly, by the eleventh century many Tibetan texts point to the existence of the practice of magical movement, especially within the traditions mentioned earlier. Although more research is needed to discover precisely how this practice originated and how it changed over time, it is clear that its roots were well established in Tibetan religious traditions over a thousand years ago, as the texts studied here attest.

The question of the origins of Bön has undergone lengthy discussions among both Tibetan and Euro-American scholars. Traditional Bön religious history claims that 18,000 years ago the buddha Tonpa Shenrab Miwoche came to a region of Central Asia known as Olmo Lungring. The teachings he gave there spread throughout Central Asia, first to the regions of Tazig and Zhang Zhung, and then to Tibet, Kashmir, India, and China. Bön histories thus claim that the Bön teachings predate Buddhism, and further that Tonpa Shenrab was actually Shakyamuni Buddha's teacher during two consecutive incarnations. In the first of these, Tonpa Shenrab was called Chime Tsugphu ("Immortal Crowned One"), and his disciple, the future Shakyamuni Buddha, was called Sangwa Dupa ("Essential Secret"). In the following life, now as Tonpa Shenrab, the future Shakyamuni Buddha was again one of his main disciples, now named Lhabu Dampa Karpo ("White Pure Son of the Gods"). Lhabu Dampa Karpo asked his teacher what he could do to help sentient beings, and Tonpa Shenrab told him that he should help the people in India who were following a wrong view. For that purpose, Tonpa Shenrab gave Lhabu Dampa Karpo an initiation so he would not forget the teachings in his future lives. In his next life he was born in India as prince of the Shakya clan and taught following the instructions previously given to him by his teacher, Tonpa Shenrab, thereby benefiting many sentient beings as the Shakyamuni Buddha. The Bön narrative thereby places the Buddha and his teachings within a larger tradition of Bön history.

Traditional Bön accounts claim that Tonpa Shenrab's main teachings were the cycles of the nine ways—sometimes called nine vehicles—and the five doors. The nine ways, being more popular, consist of four causal vehicles that concern daily life, and include medicine, astrology, divination, and funeral rites. The result vehicles are the religious disciplines relating to the sutras (such as ethical conduct and vows), tantras, and Dzogchen. Yongdzin Tenzin Namdak, widely considered the most respected contemporary scholar and lama from the Bön tradition, states that because all nine vehicles were taught by Tonpa Shenrab, they are all considered legitimate paths to enlightenment.

Bönpos themselves distinguish three kinds of Bön: early or "primitive" Bön, Yungdrung or eternal Bön, and New Bön. Early Bön is seen as an ensemble of the popular religions, similar to what Tibetan scholar Rolf Stein called "the nameless religion." That is, the religious practices that existed in Tibet before the advent of Buddhism in the seventh century. What those rituals and doctrines were is difficult to know. Yungdrung Bön is the religion that claims its origin in the Buddha Tonpa Shenrab and sees itself as a separate religion from Buddhism, even while acknowledging similarities. New Bön is a movement that surfaced in the sixteenth and seventeenth centuries, arising from the interaction and amalgamation between Yungdrung Bön and the Nyingma tradition of Buddhism, which preserves the earliest Buddhist teachings in Tibet. Today, Yungdrung Bön consists of nine vehicles, as described above. This book will not support the common misunderstanding of limiting the Bön religion to solely causal or "shamanic" vehicles, nor the equally problematic identification of all Bön practitioners with "result vehicles."

Defining Magical Movement

For years I worked to refine my understanding of the Bön magical movement by studying with Ponlob Thinley Nyima, the principal teacher at Menri Monastery in India. While pursuing the research that has resulted in this book, I met with him three times at Menri and four times in the US. It was within our conversations that we decided on the translation of "magical movement" for *trulkhor*. Khenpo Tenpa Yungdrung, current abbot of

Triten Norbutse Monastery in Nepal, says the magic refers to "the unusual effects that these movements produce in the experience of the practitioner."

In using the term "magical" to describe this practice, I am aware that it might not agree with the usual understanding in English. Partly, as H.S. Versnel writes, "our notion 'magic' is a modern-Western biased construct which does not fit representations of other cultures." Therefore, I feel that a short explanation is needed here.

The English word "magic" has many definitions, which are fairly consistent across other European languages, all of which sharing the common Latin and Greek root. However, there may be no precise equivalent outside of European contexts. Although in the past, most scholars in religion and anthropology defined magic by contrasting it with religion, this tendency is fading as our understanding of religious traditions around the globe has broadened. That is to say, religions were once seen as complex systems of ritual and philosophy in which magic had no place. This was in a time when European Christian scholars contrasted (their) religion to superstition and mythology—and to magic. Scholars today use both magic and religion in more inclusive ways, and many practices previously categorized as magical can in fact be seen as sharing a basic rationality with other human endeavors, including religion and even science and technology. As the famous science fiction author Arthur C. Clark once said, magic is "just science that we don't understand yet."

Within the context of religious studies, Jeffrey Kripal states that magic is generally understood as "a vague reliance on external forces that are never rationally defined but which can be manipulated by ritual activity." It seems clear, he continued, that "in most societies, magic forms an integral part of the sphere of religious thought and behavior, that is, with the sacred, set apart from the everyday." Furthermore, the *New Dictionary of the History of Ideas* defines magic as "the performance of acts or rites that are intended to influence a person or object," adding that "magical acts or rites are usually performed with the assistance of mystical power." This mystical power is related to an inner magic or inner transformation. We see some examples in this context such as the ability to speed-walk, reverse one's aging process, as well as the mastery over the external elements, and the feeling of a clear awareness of luminosity both inside and outside.

It is in this sense that I am using magic in "magical movement." Therefore, this yogic practice can be understood as movements that guide the manipulation of the gross and subtle bodies or dimensions (including channels, winds, and drops—subtle aspects of the mind), which can lead to internal or even mystical experiences and transformation of the practitioner. These aspects of our organism are not attested to by Western science, and so their manipulation is, to some degree, a reliance on the supernatural. We will see below, however, the science can measure some of the effects of these practices. That is the inner magic: the power that the performance of these movements can have on the experience of the practitioner and his/her state of mind.

In other words, I am using magic in a more inclusive sense of the word, which, corresponding to the above discussion, includes manipulation of external forces, alchemy, mysticism, and medicine or healing. We saw above how magical movement can bring external transformations, such as walking without touching the ground and reversing one's age, as well as more internal ones, such as desired mental experiences, which could be equated to external manipulations, alchemy and mysticism, respectively. The use as healing or medicine could be seen as a byproduct of that transformation or as one of the "unusual effects" that Khenpo Tenpa Yungdrung referred to in an earlier quote. This too can be considered magic. Magical movement can be a sufficiently advanced mind-body technology that is magical in all the ways described above.

The Body-Breath-Mind Triad

In Bön and Buddhist teachings, one's physical body, speech or energy, and mind are known as the three doors through which one practices and realizes enlightenment. Within the speech or energy realm, there is a subtle energy body that emerges both metaphorically and, for some, in actuality, as it can be experienced in these practices. This subtle energy body, also called the *vajra* body, is composed of channels and winds that run within them, providing the landscape where the mind and the physical body connect with each other. In the Tibetan yogic tradition, as described in previous chapters, there are certain practices that work specifically with the energetic or subtle body and are called "channels-and-winds," or *tsalung*, practices. Channels-and-winds is sometimes taught as a practice in itself but is often included within magical movement, in which case it is called "magical movement of channels and winds."

The Tibetan terms here translated as "channels" (*tsa*) and "winds" (*lung*) have different meanings in different contexts, and so their translations can vary, such as between medical or religious practices. There are also many variations among different texts and traditions. In Tibetan medicine, the channels—specifically the circulation channels—include those that carry not only breath and subtle winds, but also blood, and other fluids and energies that connect all aspects of the body. Therefore, *tsa*, depending on the context, is translated as "veins," "arteries," "nerves," and so forth. Here, *tsa* refers to those channels that carry *lung*, or winds. This term, similarly, has a wide range of meaning, including "air" or external wind. In the practices, *lung* does not refer to that external wind but rather to internal subtler aspects of it, such as normal breath and the subtler winds that run within the body through the meditative channels.

Channels-and-winds practices are crucial in the training and harmonizing, or balancing, of the channels and the winds of the practitioner. Put simply, in these practices, the practitioner becomes familiar with the channels first through visualization and second by using the mind to direct the winds along those channels. In this way one allows the winds to circulate through the channels more evenly in terms of the rhythm of the inhalation and exhalation and seeks a greater balance in terms of the amount and strength of the breath through the different channels. The mind rides on the wind, like a rider on a horse, and the two travel together through the pathways of the channels. As the wind circulating in the channels becomes more balanced, the channels turn increasingly pliable, allowing the winds to find their own comfortably smooth rhythm. When the wind rhythm is smooth, like a wave, the mind riding on it has a smoother ride, which reduces the tendency toward agitation. With the help of movements that guide the mind and winds into different areas, the practice brings the possibility of healing or harmonizing body, energy, and mind, or the body-energy-mind system. This is a goal of yogic practices and also a model of good health that is in line with the concept of health or well-being in Tibetan medicine.

In the Bön tradition, the principal text used for the channels-and-winds practice is the *Mother Tantra*, specifically the chapter on the "Drop or *thiklé* of the Elements." The contemporary Bönpo lama and scholar Tenzin Wangyal Rinpoche, basing his research principally on the *Mother Tantra* and his own experience, explains this kind of practice as follows:

> All experience, waking and dreaming, has an energetic basis. This vital energy or wind is called *lung* in Tibetan but is better known in the West by its Sanskrit name *prana*. The underlying structure of any experience is a precise combination of various conditions and causes. If we are able to recognize its mental, physical and energetic dynamics, then we can reproduce those experiences or alter them. This allows us to generate experiences that support spiritual practices and avoid those that are detrimental.

This is the aim of the magical movement practitioner; to engage in physical movements that guide the vital breath or wind, which in turn, guided by the mind, enables the generation of specific mental, energetic, and physical experiences.

From Patanjali, who is credited with originating Indian yoga in the second century BCE and continuing with the eleventh-century Indian saint Gorakhnath and his followers, Indian yoga texts describe how, by keeping still in a specific body posture, the mind will stop and be stable too. We also see this in many Buddhist and Bön meditation practices, where the body posture prescribed is a still lotus posture as a support to hold the mind stable. The emphasis on the mind being stable seems to be paramount for all types of yoga; however, the methods differ. According to Indologist David White, referring to classic Indian yoga, "the theory here is simple: Stop this, that stops." In other words, as we manipulate the body, the mind comes under control. White adds, however, that putting this into practice is not so simple.

In contrast to Indian styles of yoga, in magical movement the practitioner holds the breath in the way indicated in the texts, while the body moves in such a way as to guide that breath, which is guided by the mind. The body is in movement, yet the mind is able to remain still. In other words, it is not a question of "stopping," but a quite different principle. Furthermore, as we saw in the previous chapter, the magical movements themselves are seen as a tool or aid to help the mind be stable. Chinese mind-body practices, such as tai chi and qigong, share with magical movement the aspect of combining movement with particular body postures and maintaining focused attention in the midst of movement. In contrast, though, the breath is not held but rather maintained as naturally as possible, more like in Indian yogas.

According to Yongdzin Tenzin Namdak, magical movement should be used when one's meditation state is unclear, unstable, or weakened in some way. That is how early masters used them, according to the *ZZ Aural Transmission*, removing their own obstacles to abiding in their meditative state of mind. They help the practitioner, especially from the Dzogchen perspective, to regain, stabilize, or clarify the meditative state. In this way, by following instructions for the physical movements prescribed, and at the same time, holding the wind in the neutral way, the mind is allowed to rest in its own natural state. This means it is also available to rest or reside in a particular meditative state, sustained by the pervasive wind. Holding the breath in this manner during each magical movement allows the wind to pervade throughout the body. The forceful exhalation at the end, with breath and sound, helps induce the meditative state or return to the natural state of mind, which is the aim of Dzogchen practice more generally. As we saw in the previous chapter, every magical movement ends with an exhalation accompanied by the sounds of *ha* and *phat*, allowing the practitioner an opportunity to cut through any concepts that persist and then to remain more completely at rest (note that "rest" here means rest with awareness; it is not falling asleep).

Importance of Orality

In trying to understand these yogic practices we need more than just the texts. As Buddhist scholar David Gray argues, "scriptures cannot be adequately understood if orality, and the social world that gave rise to it, is not taken into account." This was made clear to me by my work with some of the major exponents of the living tradition in which these texts are embedded. The oral instructions are vital for the learning model among Tibetans. As scholar Anne Klein points out in *Path to the Middle*, the intersection between the oral and textual philosophical traditions of Tibet "creates multiple webs and layers of connections." She adds,

> Among the most important of these are the links between teacher and student, which also involve relationships between teacher and text, student and text, as well as between text and personal reflection, and which engage students and teachers with a wide variety of other texts cited in the reading, or quotes that simply come to mind in the course of reflection and conversation.

The lama, Klein continues, brings forth their "own analyses developed over a lifetime" and "adds to the reading an aura of kindliness, humor, excitement, or severity." I could not agree more. The oral explanations I received from the lamas mentioned in this study certainly were given in warmth, kindliness, humor, and excitement, with the rigorous philosophical concepts at the heart of our discussion.

I also follow Klein's inquiry into what it means to read a Tibetan text that is interwoven with a variety of oral genres, rituals, meditative techniques, and written texts, and how Westerners read or understand it. Klein notes some important differences between the Tibetan oral tradition and "the 'classical' oral characteristics noted by scholar Walter Ong." Among the genres that Klein cites, Shardza's *Commentary* is mainly a "textual commentary" or an "explanatory commentary," whereas Drugyalwa's is best understood as "instructions from experience." In my work with both Geshe Tenzin Wangyal Rinpoche on the *Commentary* and with the late Menri abbot Lungtok Tenpai Nyima on another of Shardza's texts, *Mass of Fire*, I also benefited from "word commentary," which, as its name suggests, is a commentary on "every word of a text." My work with Yongdzin Tenzin Namdak Rinpoche and most of my work with Ponlob Thinley Nyima was in effect a "commentary on the difficult points" and "instructions on the explanation." And some aspects of my work with all of them fit into the category of "essential instructions" intended to reveal "the heart of a text." All of these brought to light the beauty, depth, and richness of the *Aural Transmission of Zhang Zhung*.

The Practice and Practical Applications of Magical Movement

Among Bön exile lay and monastic communities, magical movement is primarily used to develop meditation practice. The movements also strengthen physical health and emotional stability as a secondary benefit, which is attractive to monastic and lay practitioners alike. According to Ponlob Thinley Nyima, in addition to using them to enhance their meditative experiences, Tibetan yogis and accomplished meditators practicing in caves would traditionally use magical movements to dispel bodily illness as well as mental and energetic obstacles. He notes that these yogis had no access to hospitals or other healthcare institutions, so it is through these practices that they addressed their physical and mental health. Tibetans do in fact often speak more about the physical effects of these practices. Still, upon further inquiry, while most lamas will affirm that the meditative aspect is the most crucial, they recognize that magical movement's uniqueness comes in its utilization of the body. While enhancing meditative experiences and dispelling obstacles remain the two main objectives of magical movements, at least among contemporary teachers, there is more and more an emphasis on being able to integrate those meditative experiences into everyday life and one's daily behavior.

As said before, although mainstream Western medicine has not recognized the connection between physical illness and energetic or mental obstacles, that acknowledgment exists in George Engel's bio-psycho-social model and in the emerging field of Complementary and Integrative Medicine (CIM) in ways that are similar to Asian systems of healthcare. In particular, in mind-body practices, more than a thousand studies of meditation have been reported in English and other Western languages. Over the last several years, taking impulse in this wave, I have expanded my research on these ancient practices to consider their possible practical and physical applications in a Western setting. For that purpose, I have given particular attention to the potential benefits of including magical movement as part of CIM treatments for cancer patients. In 2000, with Lorenzo Cohen, PhD, Carla Warneke, MPH, Rachel Fouladi, PhD, and M. Alma Rodriguez, MD, at the University of Texas MD Anderson Cancer Center in Houston, I conducted a randomized controlled clinical trial to determine the feasibility, acceptability, and initial efficacy of magical movements with cancer patients. For this pilot study, we designed a seven-session protocol called "Tibetan Yoga Program (TYP)," which included channels-and-winds practices from the *Mother Tantra*—in particular as described in English in Tenzin Wangyal Rinpoche's *Awakening the Sacred Body*—and the preliminary or foundational magical movement cycle described in Shardza's *Commentary*. Our hypothesis was that, through the practice of magical movement together with channels-and-winds practices, patients would be able to alleviate the mental and physical stress caused by the severe side effects of cancer treatment, such as chemotherapy or radiation.

As noted earlier, mainstream Western medicine holds a much more ironclad division between physical illness and energetic or mental obstacles, and thus it becomes difficult for most doctors to accept the connection Tibetans see between well-being and meditation, including yogic practices. Part of this difference may arise from the dichotomy between mind and body that Western thought inherited and absorbed from Cartesian dualism. In contrast, in Eastern thought, a subtle or energetic body exists which mediates between mind and body.

These studies are not necessarily done to prove one tradition right and the other wrong, but rather to prove the efficacy of meditative and yogic techniques that exist in some of these centuries-old traditions from the East, albeit in a condensed form, part of what has been called a "modern medicalization" of yoga. Studies in this light need to also acknowledge that different results might be due to differences between meditation styles. In other words, we cannot expect the same results from different meditative techniques, in the same way that we would not expect the same results from different styles of psychological therapies or from different physical therapies. Nevertheless, there are some generalities that do apply to all (or most) of them. To actually make this statement in a scientific way, we would need to research each one of them under the same protocol.

These yogic practices provide, in both realms of health and spirituality, a method of harmonizing the mind and the body by using this energetic dimension, thus harmonizing what we could call the entire mind-energy-body system. By being in touch with this mediating structure and manipulating the channels, winds, and drops through the visualization, breathings, and movements of the channels-and-winds practices and magical movements, the practitioner is expected to be able to affect not only the microcosm of the mind-energy-body system but even the macrocosm of the external universe.

Again, the connection between physical health and spiritual accomplishment is not always clearly articulated. Although these similar principles did exist in both yoga and Ayurveda, an ancient Indian medical practice, yoga was not used as part of Ayurveda, or as a healing or medical therapy. Yoga was practiced for liberation, not well-being, and so too with magical movement. What we now think of as yoga, with its emphasis of physical fitness and holistic health is a modern phenomenon, which, in particular when divorcing it from the spiritual realm, has excised classical yoga's elements of magic. I believe that research in CIM, and especially in yogic practices, may become one bridge that can build more understanding between these ancient Asian practices and mainstream Western medicine.

Shardza Tashi Gyaltsen and Magical Movement

Shardza Tashi Gyaltsen (1859–1934) emerged from a Bönpo family in eastern Tibet to become one of the most widely recognized Bönpo lamas of recent times. His vision and work as an organizer of the Bön tradition earned him a very special place in the tradition. Upon his death he achieved the rainbow body, considered the sign of highest spiritual achievement within Dzogchen schools of both Bön and Nyingma traditions.

Magical movement is only one among the many practices about which he wrote. His Five Treasuries, which is a large collection of texts, include teachings of Sutra, Tantra, and Dzogchen, and so if one studies his compositions one learns about all three paths to enlightenment. His magical movement *Commentary*—the central text for this book—is part of his *Most Profound*

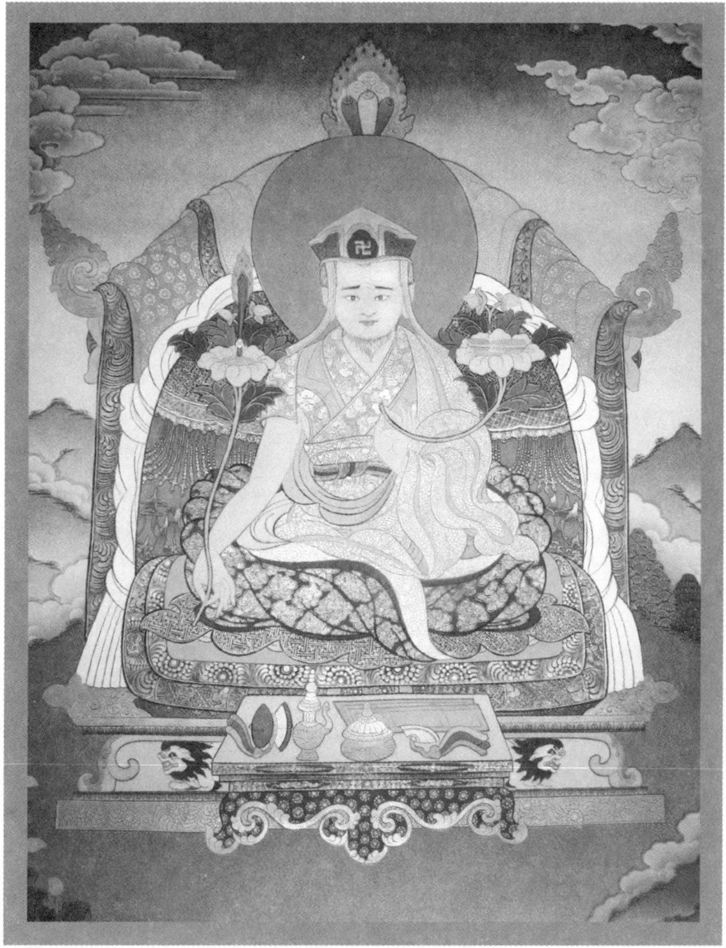

Shardza Tashi Gyaltsen

Great Sky Treasury. Shardza is somewhat controversial, in that he worked not only with Yungdrung Bön texts, but also with New Bön and Nyingma texts and masters, and so has been accused of muddying the differences between the traditions. Nonetheless, the late Menri abbot Lungtok Tenpai Nyima asserts: "Shardza did not mix; when he worked on Yundgrung Bön texts, he remained faithful to Yungdrung Bön, and when he worked on New Bön he worked within the New Bön system."

Shardza gained a wide following in part because he composed a clear system that included both the foundational and the main practices. These had not been updated since the famous thirteenth-century master Drugyalwa Yungdrung, the author of the two important Dzogchen practice manuals, *Instructions on the A* and *Experiential Transmission*, which I introduced in chapter 1. As noted earlier, *Experiential Transmission* itself was based on the eleventh- or twelfth-century text *ZZ Aural Transmission*, specifically the chapter on magical movement: *Quintessential Oral Instructions*.

Magical Movement Curricula and Practice

With respect to magical movement, Shardza systematized a full program of practice based on the tradition of magical movement from both the *ZZ Aural Transmission* and Drugyalwa's *Experiential Transmission*. He also composed a channels-and-winds liturgical prayer that is still performed today by magical movement practitioners (see appendix 2). The prayer is directed at Kuntuzangpo, who is understood as the primordial buddha and also one's natural state of mind; his name means "The All Good." It has a foundational section that includes an homage to Kuntuzangpo, securing a boundary and banishing obstacles, refuge, generation of the altruistic mind of enlightenment and a mandala offering. Its main section consists of prayers to the masters of the mind, the sign and the oral lineages beginning with Kuntuzangpo to one's own root master, and also includes meditation deities such as Takla Mebar and enlightened protectors such as Yeshe Walmo. Sometimes this prayer is sung together with a drum and bell. After experiencing the blessings of the lineage, the practitioner is advised to rest in that meditative state of mind for a moment before engaging in the yogic practices.

In another text, titled *Oral Wisdom's Main Points of Channels and Winds* (hereafter referred to as *Main Points*) Shardza delineates a one-hundred-day—or more specifically, a fourteen weeks plus two days—magical movement retreat schedule, which includes *tummo* and magical movements from *Instructions on the A* based on his *Mass of Fire* text, and *ZZ Aural Transmission* magical movements from his *Commentary*. *Main Points* is, still today, the most commonly used Bönpo text for magical movement training, In it, Shardza describes a curriculum and retreat schedule, prescribing the yogin to practice four daily sessions for a total of one hundred days. Although not specifically mentioned in *Main Points*, practitioners are expected to recite the channels-and-winds prayer at the beginning of every session.

Shardza's retreat schedule is divided into weekly periods. The first two weeks are used to perfect the gentle breathing retention, which builds up to 108 repetitions in one session. During this time, practices classified as "external foundational" are prescribed. These help the yogin familiarize with the channels, winds, and drops (the latter as a subtle expression of the mind). Following that, practices classified as "distinctive foundational" are prescribed. These include visualization of one's body as a deity, connecting to the subtle body, and applying the general foundational practices by securing a boundary, purification breaths, and a preparation for inner heat. While the external foundational practices are done for the first two weeks, the distinctive foundational practices are to be included in every session.

Then, the text instructs the practitioner, "on the morning of the fifteenth day, add the magical movement postures or body training." This third week includes the foundational magical movement cycle from the *Commentary*, and a set of fifteen magical movements from *Instructions on the A*, condensed by Drugyalwa Yungdrung from the original forty. During the fourth week, the root magical movement set from the root cycle in the *Commentary* is added to the foundational cycle, and the set of seven upper-torso purification magical movements from the cycle of forty magical movements from *Instructions on the A* is done instead of the set of fifteen magical movements condensation by Drugyalwa. Shardza also uses the sound practices, visualizations, and offerings indicated in *Instructions on the A* magical movement, which should be applied when a yogin notices an imbalance in terms of afflictions, humors, heat or cold illnesses. The four general offerings of smoke, water, burnt food, and the practice of cutting attachment to self that most Bön practitioners perform daily can be incorporated in this curriculum from the fourth week onward. Shardza exhorts here that "to validate the sessions and protect the mind, one should seal the practice with the dedication prayer and contemplation at the end."

By the end of the fourth week, the gentle breath retention training is completed, and the yogin begins with the intermediate breath retention. In this case there is no gradual accumulation, with the yogin continuing with

108 repetitions. In every session of the fifth week, the intermediate breath retention is followed by the pertinent magical movement sets. The magical movement sets added during the fifth week are the clearing obstacles from the root cycle in the *Commentary* and the set of six head purification magical movements from the cycle of forty magical movements from *Instructions on the A*.

In the sixth week, the yogin also includes the root magical movement set from the branch cycle in the *Commentary* and the set of eleven body purification magical movements from *Instructions on the A*'s cycle of forty magical movements. For the eighth and ninth weeks, the *Commentary*'s branch magical movements that clear away obstacles from the root cycle and the distinctive magical movements that clear away specific obstacles from the head, body and limbs are added, along with the set of nine lower-body purification magical movements from *Instructions on the A*'s cycle of forty magical movements. At the end of the ninth week, one finishes the training of the intermediate breath retention, bringing the winds to the different chakras and minor channels all over the subtle body.

The yogin begins the training in the forceful breath retention, described as a mass of fire of the yogic heat practice, during the tenth week. This breathing practice, also done 108 times in each session, is followed by respective magical movement sets. During this week, the distinctive magical movements that clear away common obstacles are added together with the seven leg-purification magical movements from the cycle of forty magical movements of *Instructions on the A*. Therefore, practicing in this way for the next five weeks and two days, the one hundred days are completed. Shardza concludes *Main Points* with advice on avoidances and supports, such as when it is useful to use warm clothes, receive a massage, and so forth.

The above-described sequence reflects how magical movement is practiced today in the main Bön monasteries in exile, such as Triten Norbutse in Nepal and Menri in India. This is also the case even in the present-day Tibet Autonomous Region. In particular there is a group of nuns and female practitioners practicing magical movement using Shardza's *Commentary* and *Main Points* in the Drak Yungdrung Kha nunnery in the northeastern Amdo region of Sharkhog.

Shardza's significant contribution to systematizing and clarifying the teachings makes it easier to practice and allows these wonderful traditions to continue. However, they have not been preserved in many places. I was surprised to hear that, in the northwestern Dolpo area of Nepal, where the great Yangton family lineage still continues, they do not practice magical movement, although their predecessors included axial magical movement figures. In fact, this is the lineage to which Ponlob Thinley Nyima belongs. He learned magical movement not in his home region but in Menri with Yongdzin Tenzin Namdak and His Holiness Lungtok Tenpai Nyima.

There is also a more extensive three-year curricula by Shardza, which encompasses *Main Points*. According to Ponlob Thinley Nyima, there is no specific text that mentions the curriculum in this way. However, it has been practiced in the following manner since Shardza's time: the first year includes the preliminary practices, yogic inner heat, channels-and-winds practices, and magical movement; the second year, yogic inner heat, channels-and-winds practices, and magical movement, adding nurturing from the elements practice (*chulen*); and the third year the Dzogchen practices of breakthrough and direct leap vision. This curriculum also shows the importance of the preliminary practices as a foundational base and the relation between magical movement and higher Dzogchen practices.

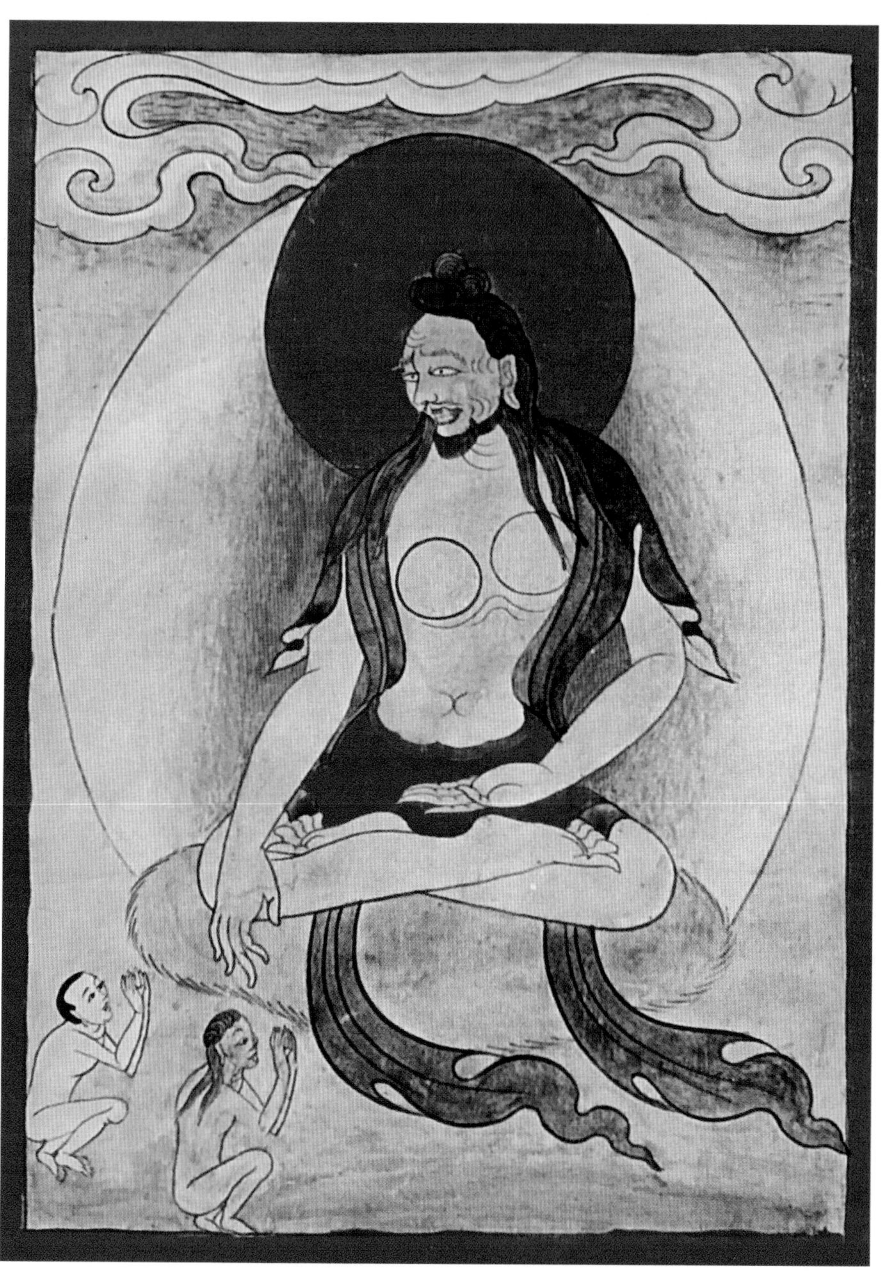

Pongyal Tsenpo

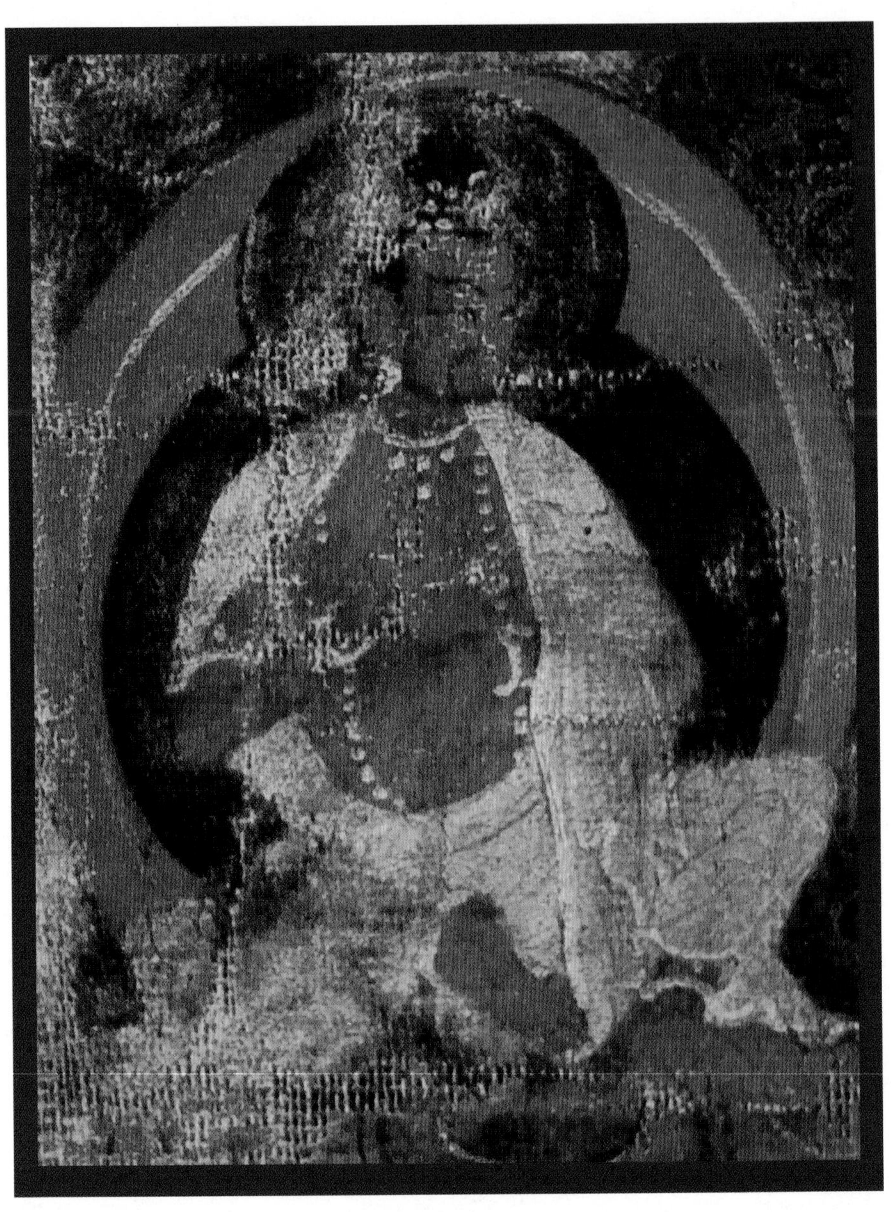

Togme Shigpo

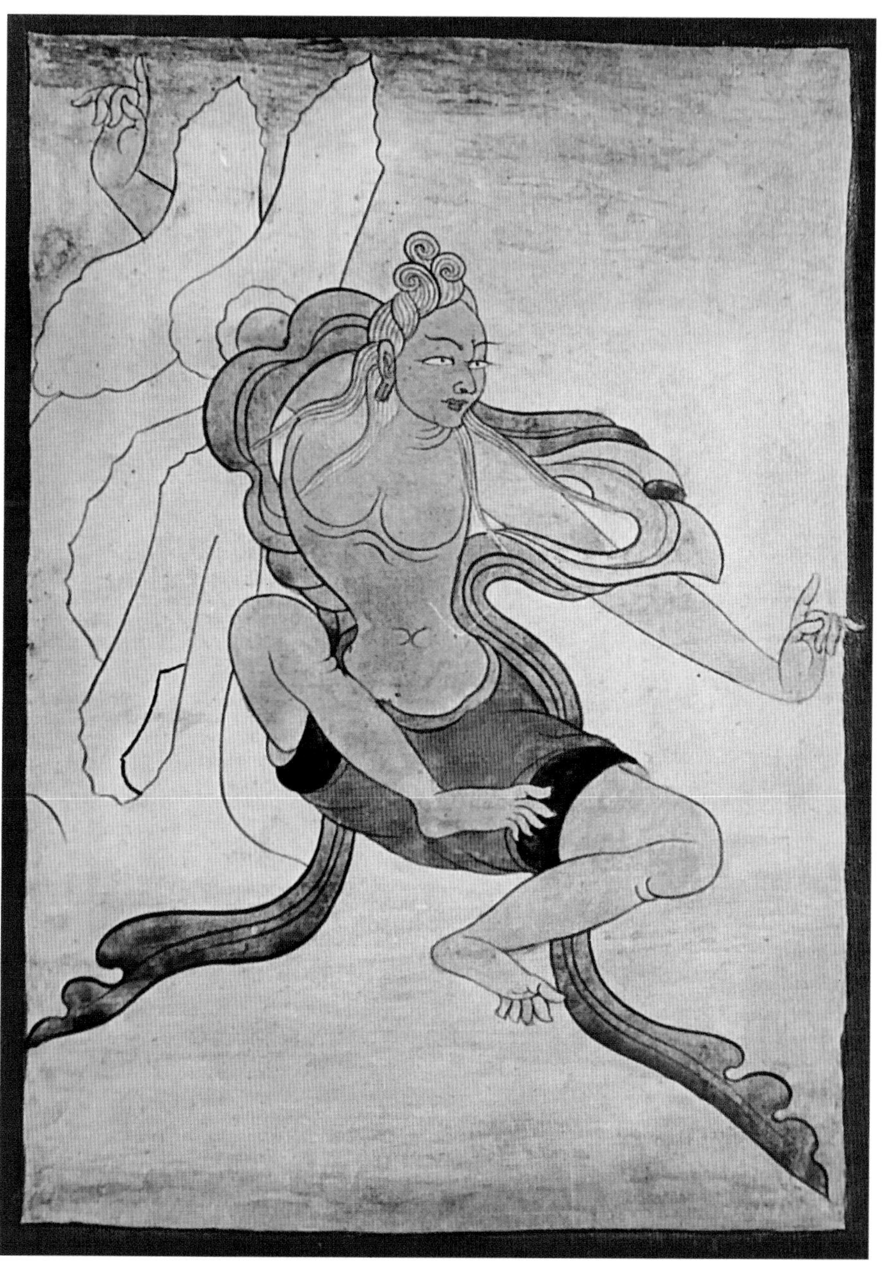

Lhundrub Muthur

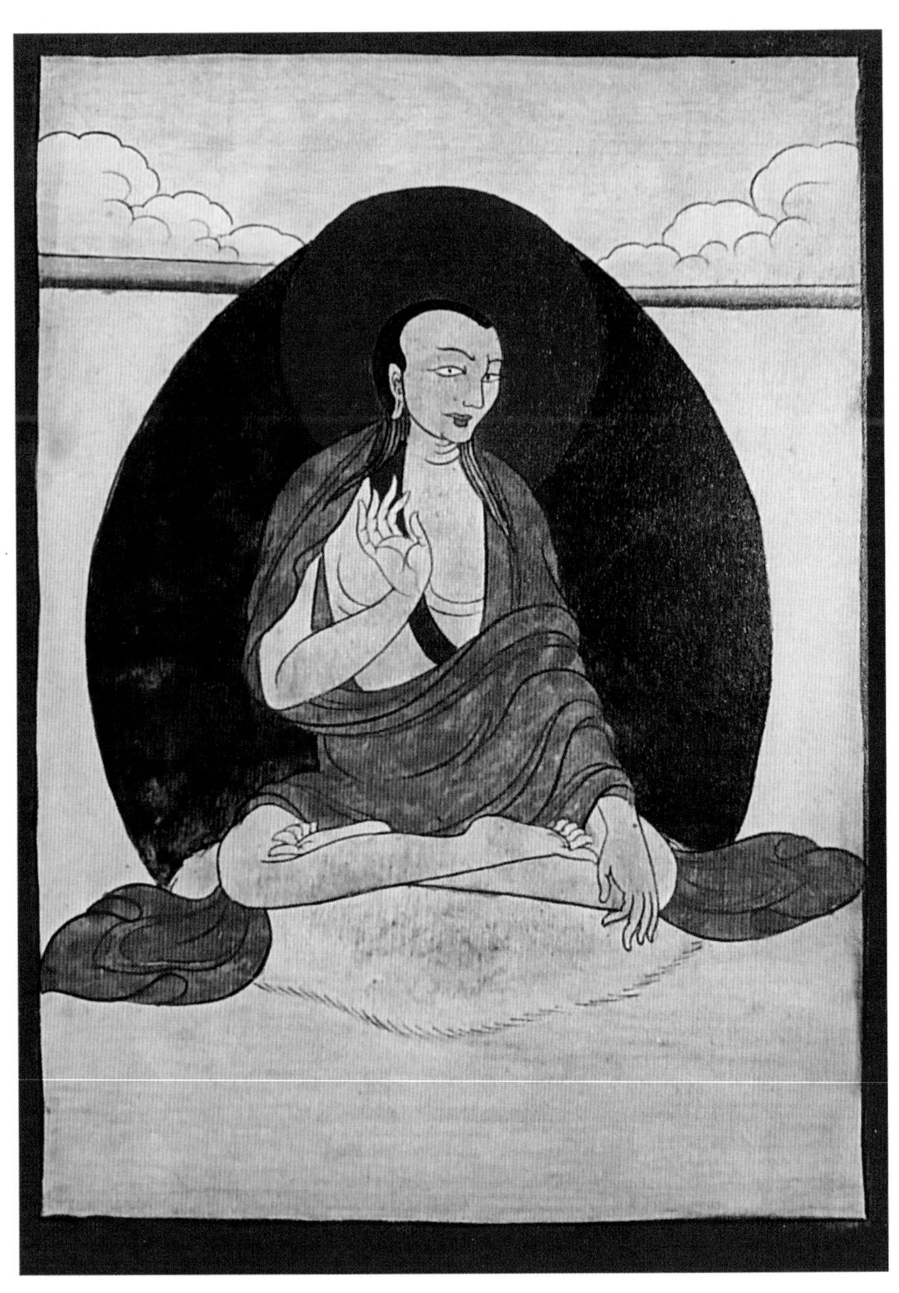

Orgom Kundul

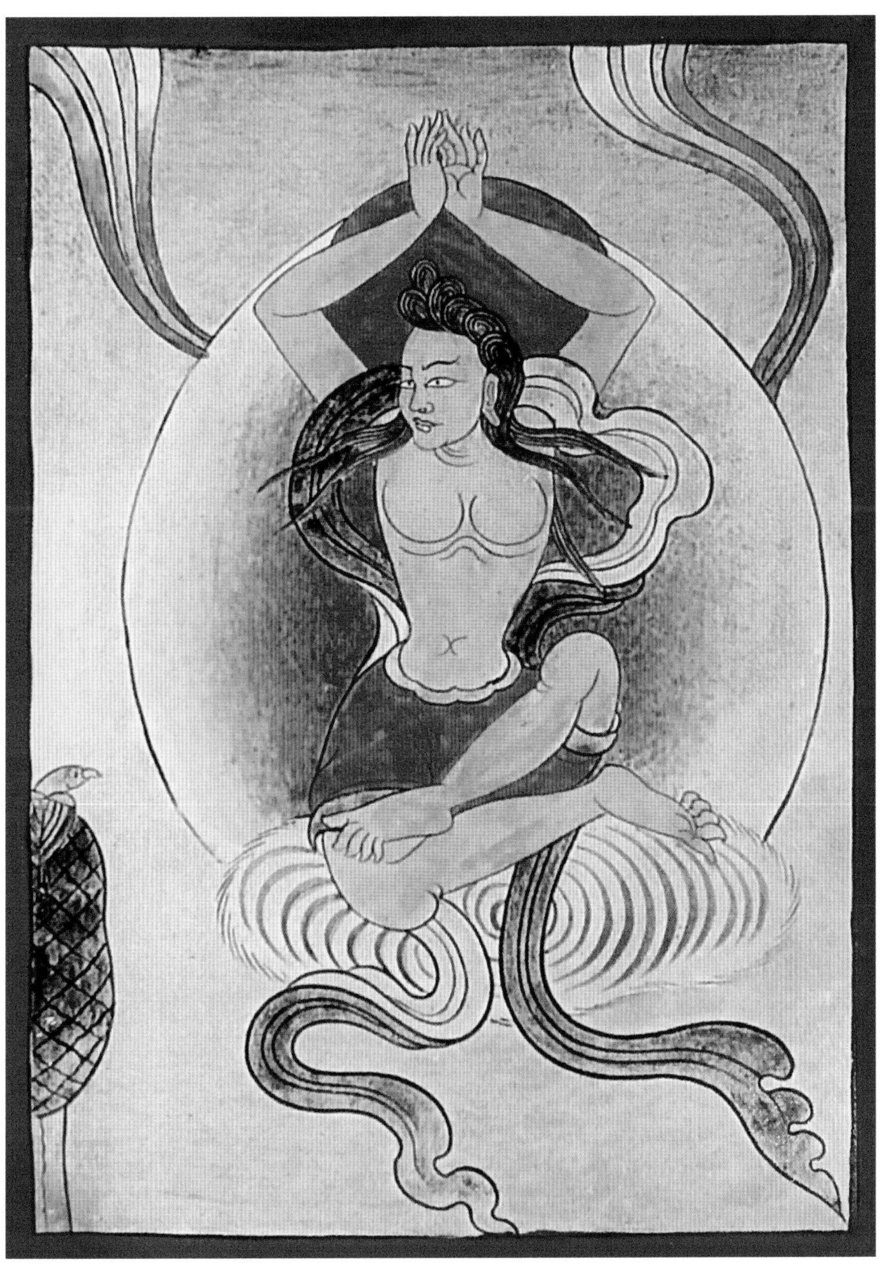

Yangton Chenpo

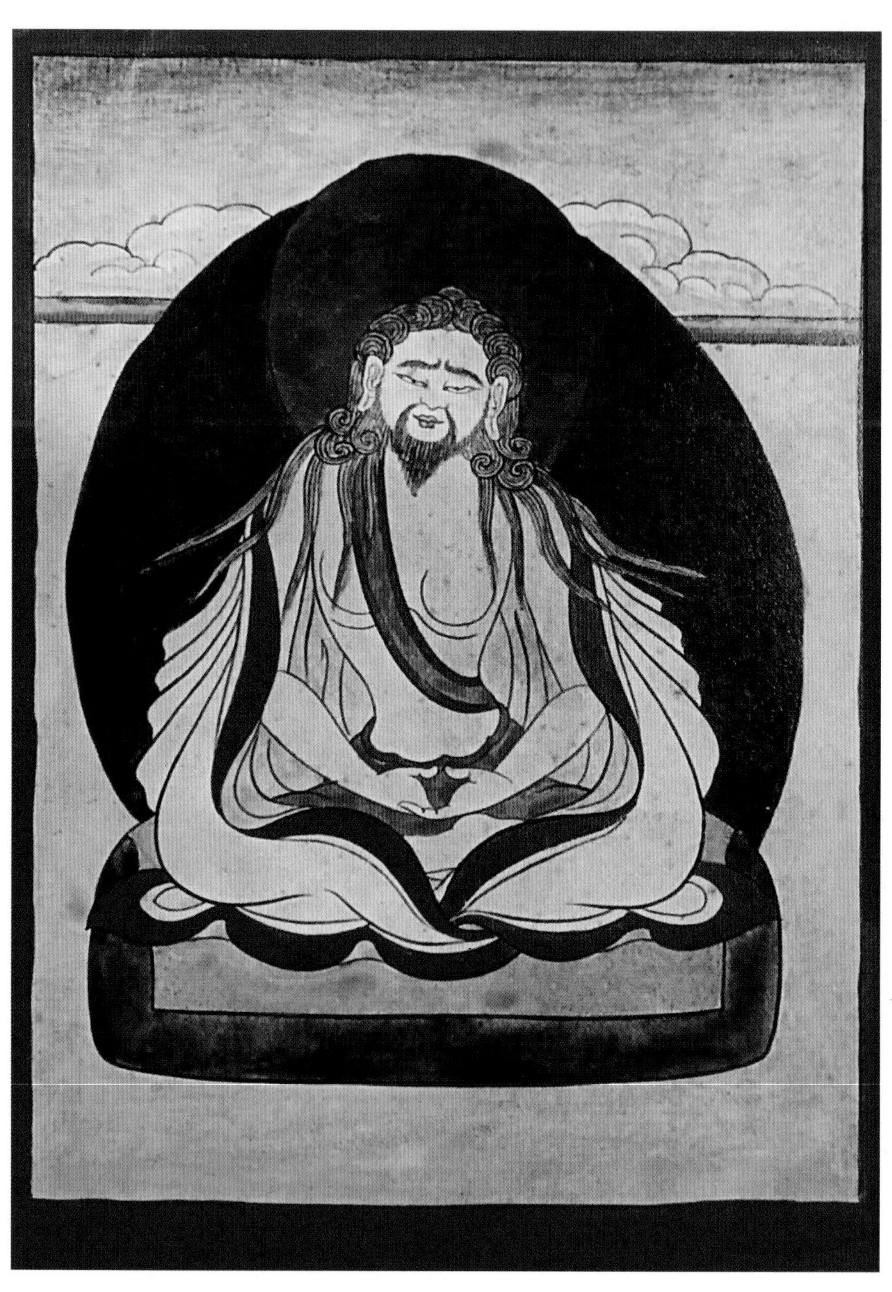

Bumje Ö

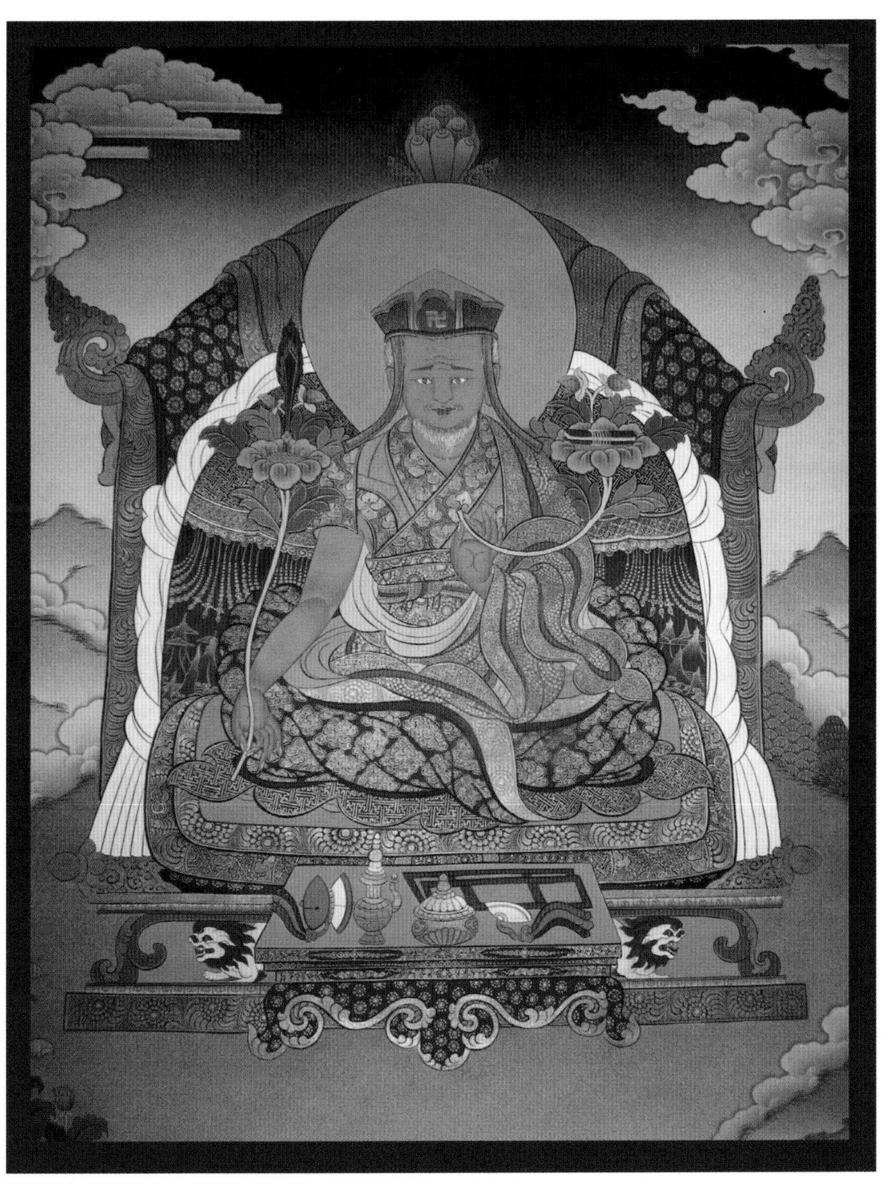

Shardza Tashi Gyaltsen

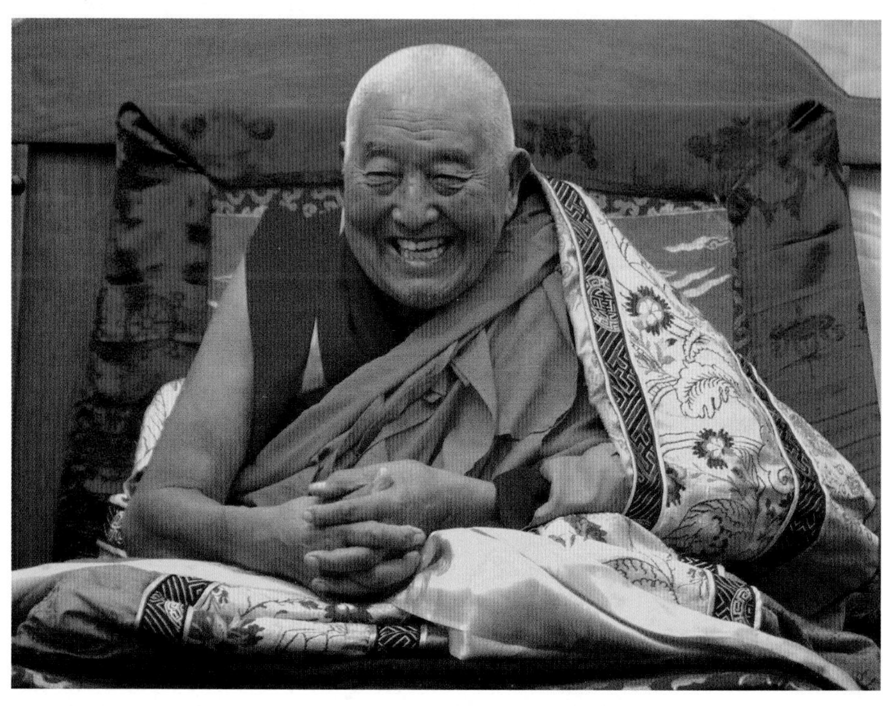

Yongdzin Tenzin Namdak

CHAPTER FOUR

Moving Forward

Magical Movement Reaches the West

NEARLY A CENTURY after Shardza's *Commentary*, there seems to be a growing interest for the Tibetan physical yogas in the West. In the last few years alone, *Yoga Journal* has published three articles on the topic: the first on the different types of Tibetan yogas that have come to the US, a second one on the magical movement paintings of the Lhasa Naga Temple—the so-called the secret temple of the Dalai Lamas behind the famous Potala Palace—and a third on the benefits of magical movement with cancer patients. More will surely follow.

There are many kinds of magical movement practices in the different Tibetan traditions, and they are slowly being made known to us. The Yantra Yoga that is taught in Namkhai Norbu Rinpoche's Dzogchen Community is based on the Tibetan text *Union of Sun and Moon*, which is credited to the eighth-century Tibetan master Vairocana. There are a number of books published on Yantra Yoga and there is also an instructional video available containing the first eight movements, which aim to purify one's breath and are considered to be preparatory movements. The magical movement that is taught in Tenzin Wangyal Rinpoche's Ligmincha Institute comes from two separate, related lineages of texts: *Quintessential Oral Instructions* and Shardza's *Commentary*, and *Instructions on the A*. There is also Tibetan Heart Yoga, taught by Geshe Michael Roach and his students, a modern system based on Tsongkhapa's commentary on the *Six Yogas of Naropa*.

Tenzin Wangyal Rinpoche, through his Ligmincha International, teaches the channels-and-winds practices from the *Mother Tantra*, specifically from the chapter known as the "*Thiklé* of the Elements," and his wonderful book in English: *Awakening the Sacred Body*. This practice familiarizes the practitioner with the five kinds of winds, and Rinpoche has done a number of YouTube videos. There is also an online course on these practices through Ligmincha Learning. Magical movement is taught at Ligmincha International based on both *ZZ Aural Transmission* and *Instructions on the A*. However, the hundred-day curriculum created by Shardza that includes both lineages of magical movements is almost impossible to do in a Western setting. In lieu of that, a curriculum consisting of a series of four-to-five-day intensive retreats was created to accommodate the teachings.

Ligmincha *Trulkhor* Training Course

Tenzin Wangyal Rinpoche is quite aware of the problem of the lack of context and continuity that Westerners sometimes face when training in meditative practices, not to mention the tendency to skip over the foundational practices and jump directly to more advanced practices. At Ligmincha International he continues to design ways to transmit his tradition to Western practitioners by taking into account the conditions of body, speech and mind, and creating training courses accordingly.

In 2001, Tenzin Wangyal Rinpoche asked me to teach a formal magical movement training course at Ligmincha's main site, Serenity Ridge, near Charlottesville, Virginia. This course was composed of five five-day retreats spanning over two years. The first retreat included the channels-and-winds practices from the *Mother Tantra*, the preparatory breathing techniques to magical movement (with the "basket" or gentle retention, the first of three methods for retaining the breath) mentioned in the *Commentary* and expanded by Shardza in his *Mass of Fire*, and the first two magical movement sets from the *Commentary*. In each of the two subsequent retreats, two more magical movement sets were taught and practiced, along with the "vase" or intermediate breath retention for the preparatory breaths, the second method. In the fourth retreat, the seventh and final set was taught, together with instruction of the "mass of fire" or forceful method of the retention of the breath, although this method is to be done with caution and only when one is very familiar with reaching to 108 repetitions of the vase retention. This leaves the fifth and last retreat to the complete practice of all the movements, breathings, and focusings of the mind, as well as to have private interviews with each trainee on what the next steps are for those with intentions of sharing the practices with others.

The main purpose of this course is to offer an opportunity to both those who are seriously interested in beginning, as well as to those eager to deepen their understanding of, magical movement. Some of the participants are long-time meditators with a need for a more embodied practice, while others come from other yoga traditions, and yet others are new to any contemplative practice. The time between retreats allows the participants to practice and study what was learned so as to apply it in the next level. A secondary purpose is to train future instructors who will be able to share with others the benefits of this practice. Therefore, this training is one of the prerequisites for a magical movement instructor in this tradition.

Regardless of motivation, Tenzin Wangyal Rinpoche presents the teaching as a practice to be integrated with one's daily life, as he says:

> *Trulkhor* is a wonderful daily practice, especially to control and handle the stress of our modern life in society. It has the power to balance the energies of mind and body and it also helps enormously to support one's meditation practices.

Tenzin Wangyal Rinpoche has taught in the West for almost thirty years and is very aware of the lifestyle of Western practitioners. With that in mind, in 2007, he felt there was a need for a simpler magical movement practice for Ligmincha International practitioners. He coordinated an effort to design an abridged version of the forty magical movements from *Instructions on the A* into fifteen movements—or sixteen if we add the foundational movement. Informally we call it the Ligmincha 16. Based on it, I wrote *Tibetan Yoga for Health & Well-Being*, explaining also the process of the abridged version as well as its differences with Drugyalwa's condensation of the forty movements. And, through Ligmincha International, we created another, simpler, magical movement training. This training is done in three four-day retreats, where participants learn the different breathings, the channels-and-winds movements relating to the five kinds of breaths, and the sixteen magical movements. Wisdom Experience now has an introductory online course for Tibetan Yoga that includes six of these sixteen movements. After those three retreats, some are invited to a one-year theoretical/practical training to be able to instruct others. In fact, as I am concluding this book, we have two groups in that training—one in the US and one in Europe.

From Dharma to Medicine: Complementary and Integrative Medicine (CIM) applications with cancer patients

> *I believe that spirituality and science are complementary but different investigative approaches with the same goal of seeking the truth. In this, there is much each may learn from the other, and together they may contribute to expanding the horizon of human knowledge and wisdom.*
>
> H. H. the XIV Dalai Lama

As mentioned in earlier chapters, the twentieth century also brought the medicalization of different kinds of yoga and contemplative practices. His Holiness the Dalai Lama had been an inspiration for me, particularly in the integration of spirituality and healthcare, and Tenzin Wangyal Rinpoche has long had an interest in the healing capacity of meditative practices from his tradition, as well as in finding ways of quantifying and verifying their effects. In the early 1990s, as a Rockefeller Fellow at Rice University, he began conversations with Ellen Gritz, PhD, chair of the Department of Behavioral Science at the University of Texas MD Anderson Cancer Center. That conversation lay dormant like a stored seed for a few years. In 2000, I met with Lorenzo Cohen, an associate professor in that department who later became the director of the Integrative Medicine Program at that institution. He asked me to create a Tibetan yoga program for cancer patients. When I reviewed it with Yongdzin Tenzin Namdak and Tenzin Wangyal Rinpoche in the summer of 2000, they were extremely supportive, and so I decided to go forward with this project. The seed had begun to germinate.

Tenzin Rinpoche's open-mindedness and support were crucial for the development of this program at MD Anderson. Viewing the main goals of magical movement as dispelling mental and physical obstacles, the enhancing of meditative practice, and their integration into daily life, the MD Anderson-Ligmincha team began a study applying a seven-week Tibetan yoga program (TYP) with lymphoma patients. The movements chosen were simple, and yet they constituted complete cycles: the five external channels-and-winds movements from the *Mother Tantra* and foundational cycle magical movements from Shardza's *Commentary*. Tenzin Rinpoche reviewed the TYP intervention before patient recruitment began.

The First Study

In the first study of Tibetan yoga at MD Anderson Cancer Center, thirty-nine lymphoma patients were randomly assigned to be either in a Tibetan yoga intervention group or in a waitlisted control group. The intervention group received the seven-week TYP, while the waitlisted control group did not at that time. Measurements were taken of both groups to compare any significant health or behavior changes between participants of one group and the other. In order to be eligible, lymphoma patients had to be currently undergoing treatment or had to have concluded treatment, consisting mostly of radiation and/or chemotherapy, within the past twelve months. There was an even distribution of severity of disease between the two groups among those who were under active treatment. In addition, fifteen patients in each group were not receiving treatment for their lymphoma at the time of the study.

Patients of both groups completed self-reported evaluations at baseline (i.e., before they began the program) as well as one week, one month, and three months after the seven-week program. The whole study took almost a full year to complete, including patient recruitment at the lymphoma clinic at MD Anderson and various seven-week Tibetan yoga interventions at Place of Wellness, the clinic for CIM therapies at MD Anderson. We began the seven-week sessions after each recruitment cycle, which allowed us to teach the classes to four to nine people in each session.

Results

Eighty-nine percent of Tibetan yoga participants completed at least two to three yoga sessions; 58 percent completed at least five sessions. Overall, the results indicated that the Tibetan yoga program was feasible and well-liked by the patients. The majority of participants indicated that the program was "a little" or "definitely" beneficial, with no one indicating "not beneficial," and they continued practicing at least once a week after the conclusion of the study, with many continuing to practice twice a week or more. It is worthwhile to mention that none of the patients involved in these studies had any previous knowledge of even the existence of channels-and-winds practices or magical movement, and the majority of the patients had never engaged in any other meditative or yoga practice before.

Patients in the Tibetan yoga group reported significantly lower sleep disturbance scores during the follow-up period than did the patients in the control group. This included better subjective sleep quality, faster sleep latency (i.e., from the moment one decides to sleep until when one actually falls asleep), sleep duration, and less use of sleep medications. Improving sleep quality in a cancer population may be particularly salient, as sleep is crucial for recovery. Fatigue and sleep disturbances are common problems for patients with cancer. This research focused on behavioral changes and quality-of-life improvement. In the future, it is possible that changes in immune function, blood pressure, and eventually even disease progression could be measured.

Dr. Cohen, the principal investigator of the study, was optimistic about the results. "Theoretically, if the Tibetan Yoga intervention is found to decrease the patient's stress level, it could, therefore, have an impact on their immune system," he said. "There is evidence to suggest that stress suppresses cell-mediated immunity, a component of the immune system involved in tumor surveillance. Yoga might also have an impact on patients' hormonal activity."

As the investigators of this study acknowledged, although research into the efficacy and mechanisms of yoga is in its beginning stages, the findings reported to date are supportive and, along with our finding of improved sleep, suggest that the health effects of yoga in cancer patients should be explored further. The benefits that have been documented and the potential impact of these benefits on the lingering psychologic and physical effects of cancer are important enough to warrant the further study of developing such programs for cancer patients.

Subsequent Studies

The clinical study mentioned above showed encouraging signs for the positive effect that magical movement might have with cancer patients, and was published in *Cancer*, the journal of the American Cancer Society, in 2004. The fact that the first study was published in a mainstream medical journal such as *Cancer* was a promising sign for the inclusion of Tibetan practices within CIM clinical services and research possibilities.

This motivated us to do a second study, now examining the benefits of this Tibetan yoga program on both psychological and physiological (immune and hormone function) outcomes in women with breast cancer. This was a slightly larger study, with fifty-nine participants with eligibility factors similar to the lymphoma study, but now in a population that is much larger: women with breast cancer. It followed the same seven-week TYP, as well as the self-reported forms of measurement and structure of assessment. These pilot programs were among the few studies of yoga in a cancer patient population and the only scientific studies of magical movement in any population. One important thing we noticed in this second pilot study was that from the women in the Tibetan yoga group, those receiving chemotherapy had more improvements than those undergoing radiation.

With that precedent and results, in 2006, we were very glad to receive a large National Cancer Institute grant from the US National Institutes of Health (NIH) to support a five-year randomized trial to examine a Tibetan yoga intervention for women with breast cancer undergoing chemotherapy. One of the publications from this study, in *Cancer* (January 2018), detailed how those who practiced more than twice a week had long-term benefits. This was useful information for the clinicians in integrative medicine to be able to recommend these practices with an appropriate "dose."

In addition, in 2015 we published, in *Psycho-Oncology*, a single-arm trial of a simpler Tibetan yoga intervention for people with lung cancer and their caregivers, which helped not only the patient, but also the caregiver, and improved their relationship. And in 2013, also in *Psycho-Oncology*, we published a randomized trial using a Tibetan sound meditation (TSM) intervention for women with breast cancer that had experienced cognitive deficiencies due to the chemotherapy, what is sometimes called "chemo-brain." As the field of neuroscience and contemplative practices unfolds, this intervention showed that these women could recuperate short-term memory as well as improve cognitive function. You can see the citations for these studies in the bibliography.

Looking to the Future

These studies were unique in their collaboration between representatives of the Western biomedical and behavioral sciences communities and representatives of the Bön tradition.

Participants were taught this program as a progressive didactic and experiential set of classes with the aim of helping the patient incorporate these techniques into their everyday lives. From the Tibetan tradition perspective, these practices clear away obstacles and enhance one's meditative state of mind in order to incorporate that cultivated meditative state of mind into everyday behavior. These exercises help participants not only to regulate their breath, but also to calm their mind, and help in clearing physical, emotional, and mental obstacles. The meditative concentration techniques help to harness the calmness of mind toward self-observation and use the breathing exercises to clear away obstacles.

In some of our meetings, attended by both Dr. Lorenzo Cohen and Tenzin Wangyal Rinpoche, we began exploring different research tools that could assess not only what is interesting from the biomedical and behavioral scientific approaches, but also whether the benefits mentioned in the magical movement texts can actually be proven to be true outcomes for these cancer patients. Rinpoche expressed that the main benefit he would like to see is improvement in openheartedness, to which Dr. Cohen replied that there were no measurements yet, but he agreed that it would be a wonderful result to aim for.

In addition, dialoguing with the Tibetan medical practitioner Dr. Yeshe

Dhonden, former physician to His Holiness the Dalai Lama, we discussed the possibility of including Tibetan medical assessments to a sub-group of the breast cancer population of the study. These Tibetan experts would bring in traditional Tibetan medical categories such as the humors. In that way, one could also evaluate, according to patients' humoral constitution, to whom the magical movements would be more beneficial, or detrimental, and perhaps, indicating different movements for different patients. Although we have not been able to include those Tibetan medicine aspects yet, I consider this kind of interaction and mutual participation an important step toward a more integrative model of applying Tibetan traditional modalities of healing together with Western science and research methods.

This work has not only put Western scientific ideas on medical research in dialogue with Tibetan spiritual practice; it has also allowed for changes in both sides toward finding a sound methodological research, and more importantly, bringing some benefit to people with cancer and their families.

Furthermore, this opens the possibility to other populations beyond those suffering from cancer, including healthy individuals who want to have better overall health. As these studies continue, all of us who participate in them are constantly being reshaped, which in turn reshapes the fields in which we work, such as integrative medicine.

I hope that these Tibetan yoga research studies contribute in a small way to the bigger picture of the exploration of a new medicine that includes science and spirituality, highlighting the importance of mind-body practices as part of a healthy lifestyle, not only for the ultimate truth of healing (i.e., enlightenment) but also toward the conventional truth of the bio-psycho-social-spiritual or mind-energy-body as optimal health. And ultimately, to openheartedness.

APPENDIX 1

Shardza's *Commentary*

[321] ༄༅། ཡང་ཟབ་ནམ་མཁའ་མཛོད་ཆེན་ལས། སྙན་
བརྒྱུད་རྩ་རླུང་འཁྲུལ་འཁོར་བཞུགས་སོ།
[322] ཀུན་ཏུ་བཟང་པོ་ཕྱི་ནང་བར་ཆོད་སེལ་ལ་ཕྱག་
འཚལ་ལོ། །སྙན་བརྒྱུད་ཀྱི་རྩ་རླུང་འཁྲུལ་འཁོར་འདི་
ལ་འཁྲུལ་འཁོར་ཞལ་ཤེས་ལས། རླུང་གིས་དུག་ཕྱུང་རྩ་
འདུལ་བསྟན་པ་ལ། རྩུབ་རླུང་གཡས་ནས་ཕྱི་རུ་དྲག་ཏུ་
འབུད།། རྔུབས་རླུང་གཡོན་ནས་རིང་དུ་དལ་གྱིས་བརྔུབ།།
ཞེས་པ་ནི་རླུང་དུག་ཕྱུང་བའི་ཚུལ་ཡིན་ཏེ་བླ་མའི་ཞལ་
ལས་ཤེས། མ་ནིང་རང་ལུས་ཀུན་ལ་ཁྱབ་པར་བཟུང་།།
ཞེས་པ་ནི་དངོས་གཞིའི་རླུང་ཡིན་ཏེ།

The channels-and-winds magical movement from the *Aural Transmission of Zhang Zhung*, in *Most Profound Great Sky Treasury*

Homage and Introduction

Homage to Kuntuzangpo, who clears the outer and inner obstacles. As for these channels-and-winds magical movements of the aural tradition of Zhang Zhung, *Quintessential Oral Instructions* states:

> Regarding the teaching on training the channels and extracting the poisons of the wind: forcefully expel the coarse wind through the right channel. Inhale long and slow through the left channel.

This is a method for extracting the poisons of the wind. Understand these from the teachings of a lama. *Quintessential Oral Instructions* continues:

> Hold the neutral wind in your entire body. This is the actual wind practice.

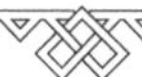

འཇམ་རླུང་། བར་རླུང་། [323]རྩུབ་རླུང་ངམ་དྲག་རླུང་
དང་གསུམ་ཡིན་ཞིང་། འཇམ་རྩུབ་བར་མ་གསུམ་ཀ་ལ་
ཐུན་བཞི་བཞིར་རླུང་ཁུག་པ་བརྒྱ་དང་བརྒྱད་རེ་ཐོན་
པའི་མཇུག་ཏུ་འཁྲུལ་འཁོར་བྱ་བ་ལ། སྔོན་འགྲོ། རྩ་བ།
ཡན་ལག །བྱེ་བྲག་དང་བཞི་ཡོད་དོ། སྔོན་འགྲོ་ལ་དྲུག་ཏུ་
བཤད་ཀྱང་ཞལ་ཤེས་ལས། མགོ་སྦྱངས། རྐང་སྦྱངས། ལག་
སྦྱངས། སྟོད་སྦྱངས། སྨད་སྦྱངས་དང་ལྔ་ལ་འདུས་པའི།

The gentle wind retention, the intermediate wind retention, and the rough wind or forceful wind retention are the three wind-retention practices. All three of the gentle, rough, and intermediate practices should be performed for 108 respirations in each of four sessions, and at the end of expelling the wind perform the magical movements. Those movements have four cycles: foundation, root, branch, and distinctive movements.

Foundational Cycle

Even though the foundational movements are explained as being six, in my own oral instructions they are condensed into five: "purification of the head," "purification of the legs," "purification of the arms," "purification of the torso," and "purification of the lower part of the body."

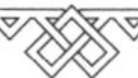

དང་པོ་མགོ་སྦྲེངས་ནི། སྐྱིལ་ཀྲུང་བྱ་ལ་ལག་པ་གཉིས་ཀྱིས་[324]མགོ་དང་ལུས་གཡས་དང་གཡོན་དང་མདུན་ཕྱོགས་གསུམ་ནས་མར་སྦྱུག་པ་ལན་རེ་བྱ། ནད་གདོན་སྡིག་སྒྲིབ་འདོན་ཕྱིར་ཧ་སྒྲ་དང་། འཁོར་བ་དོང་ནས་སྤྲུགས་ཏེ་སེམས་ཅན་ཐམས་ཅད་སངས་རྒྱས་པར་བསམ་ལ་ཕཊ༔སྒྲ་འདོན་པ་ནི་འཁྲུལ་འཁོར་ཀུན་ལ་འདྲེས་སོ།

1. Purification of the Head

Sitting cross-legged, with your two hands sweep downward from the head to the body in three directions: right, left, and directly in front, one time each. In order to expel illnesses, demons, negativities, and obscurations, sound *ha* and shake cyclic existence from its depths by shaking the body and limbs; while reflecting that all sentient beings are buddhas, pronounce the sound *phat*: apply these two practices to all the magical movements.

།གཉིས་པ་རྐང་སྦྱངས་ནི། རྐང་པ་གཉིས་བརྐྱང་ལ་ལག་
སོར་གཡོན་གྱིས་རྐེད་པར་འབྱུད་ཅིང་ལག་པ་གཡས་
ཀྱིས་ལུས་གཡས་ཕྱོགས་ནས་རྐང་པ་གཡས་པ་མར་དྲག་
ཏུ་ཐུག་ནས་རྐང་པའི་སོར་མོ་རྣམས་བཟུང་ལ་སྦྲུགས་
པ་ལན་བདུན་བྱ། གཡོན་ཡང་དེ་བཞིན་འགྲེས། གསུམ་པ་
ལག་སྦྱངས་ནི། སྐྱིལ་ཀྲུང་བྱ་ལ་ལག་པ་གཡས་པའི་མཐེ་
བོང་གི་སྲིན་མཛུབ་མནན་ཏེ་ཁུ་ཚུར་བཅངས་པ་རྡོ་རྗེ་
ཁུ་ཚུར་ཟེར་བའི་ཁུ་ཚུར་མཆན་ཁུང་ལ་རེག་ཙམ་གྱི་ཕར་
[325]དྲག་ཏུ་བརྐྱང་ལ་སོར་མོ་བཀྲོལ་བ་དེ་ལྟར་ལན་
བདུན་བྱ། གཡོན་ཡང་དེ་བཞིན་འགྲེས།

2. Purification of the Legs

Sitting with both legs extended, the fingers of your left hand hold your waist, and then with your right hand vigorously sweep the right side of your body all the way to the toes. Then, holding the tips of the toes, shake. Do this seven times. Apply this practice in a similar manner to the left side.

3. Purification of the Arms

Sitting cross-legged, with the thumb of your right hand press the base of the ring finger. Making a fist, called a *vajra* fist, gently touch it to your armpit; then vigorously extend it outward while releasing the fingers. Do this seven times. Apply this practice in a similar manner to the left side.

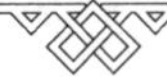

བཞི་པ་སྟོད་སྦྱངས་ནི། སྐྱིལ་ཀྲུང་བྱ་ལ་ལག་པ་གཉིས་ཀྱི་ལག་ངར་གཉིས་གཤིབས་ཏེ་ལག་མཐིལ་གཉིས་ས་ལ་བསྟན་ལ་མདུན་དུ་ཕར་བརྒྱང་ཚུར་བཀུག་ལག་མགོ་བྲང་ལ་རེག་པ་ལན་བདུན་བྱས་པའི་རྗེས་སུ། ལུས་ཀུན་སྤྲུགས་པ་དང་མཉམ་དུ་ཧ་སྒྲ་ཐེབས་གསུམ་འདོན། ལྔ་པ་སྨད་སྦྱངས་ནི། རྐང་པ་གཉིས་བརྐྱང་ལ་ལག་གཉིས་ཀྱིས་མཉམ་དུ་ལུས་སྟོད་ནས་མར་འཕུར་བྱུག་བྱེད་ཅིང་གཟུགས་བཞི་སྤྲུགས་བརྐྱང་ལན་བདུན་བྱས་རྗེས་ཧ་དང་ཕཊ༔ སྒྲ་འདོན་པ་ཀུན་ལ་འགྲེས་སོ།

4. Purification of the Upper Torso

Sitting cross-legged, bring your two arms parallel. With the two palms facing the ground, extend them in front and then bend them back inward, touching the chest with the top of the hand. After doing this seven times, simultaneously shake the entire body and expel breath using the sound *ha* three times, followed by one *phat*.

5. Purification of the Lower Body

Sitting with both legs extended, with both hands together, massage from the top of the body downward with a sweeping motion, and then extend and shake the four limbs seven times.

Expel using the sounds *ha* and *phat*, applying this to each magical movement.

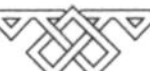

།སྔོན་འགྲོའི་འཁྲུལ་འཁོར་ཡོན་ཏན་ནི། འཁྲུལ་འཁོར་
ཞལ་ཤེས་ལས། རྩ་རླུང་ཆ་སྙོམས་རྩའི་སྒྲུབས་སེལ་བར་
[326]བྱེད། འབྱུང་བཞི་ཆ་སྙོམས་ཕུང་པོ་གནད་དུ་ཚུད།།
རིག་པ་དྭངས་ཤིང་རླུང་གི་བྱེ་བྲག་ཕྱེད། དཔོན་རྒྱལ་
བཙན་པོའི་དགོངས་པའོ། །ཞེས་སོ། ༔ །རྩ་བའི་འཁྲུལ་
འཁོར་ལ། རྩ་བ་དྲུག་དང་། གེགས་སེལ་དྲུག་གོ །རྩ་བ་
དྲུག་ནི། ཞི་སྣང་གྱད་ཀྱི་ཐོ་བརྡེག །གཏི་སྨུག་ཡེ་ཤེས་
སྐར་ཁྱུང་། ང་རྒྱལ་འཁོར་ལོ་བཞི་སྒྲིལ། འདོད་ཆགས་རྒྱ་
མདུད་ཟུར་དཀྲོལ། ཕྲག་དོག་དར་ལྕེ་གྱེན་སྐྱུགས། །ཁྱིང་
ཁོད་སྟག་མོ་མཆོང་སྟབས་སོ།

Benefits

Regarding the benefits of the foundational magical movements, *Quintessential Oral Instructions* states:

> The channels and winds are balanced, and the interior of the channels are cleared. The four elements are balanced, and the vital points of the aggregates of the body are penetrated, making the body function well. Awareness is lucid and the flow of each of the distinct winds is freed. These are the exalted perspectives of Pongyal Tsenpo.

Root Cycle (Root Magical Movement Set)

As for the root magical movements, they are the six root movements and the six that clear obstacles. The six root movements are "striking the athlete's hammer to overcome hatred," "skylight of primordial wisdom to overcome delusion," "rolling the four limbs like wheels to overcome pride," "loosening the corner of the braided knot to overcome desire," "waving the silk tassel upward to overcome jealousy," and "the stance of a tigress's leap to overcome drowsiness and agitation."

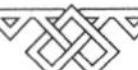

།དྲུག་པ་ཞི་སྡང་གྱད་ཀྱི་ཐོ་བརྡེག་ནི། ལག་པ་གཉིས་ལྷག་
ཁུང་དུ་སོར་མོ་བསྣོལ་ནས་འཁྱུད། པུས་མོ་གཉིས་ས་ལ་
བཙུགས་ནས་རྐང་པའི་བོལ་ཚིག་གཉིས་རྒྱབ་ཏུ་བསྣོལ་ཏེ།
ལྡིད་རྣམས་པུས་མོར་བཀལ་ལ་རྐེད་པ་བསྲང་ཞིང་།
མཇིང་པ་རྒྱབ་[327]ཏུ་དགྱེད་ཅིང་ནང་དུ་བཀུག་པའི་
གྲུ་མོ་གཉིས་པུས་མོ་གཉིས་ལ་རེག་པ་དེ་འདྲ་ལན་བདུན་
བྱ། བདུན་པ་གཏི་མུག་ཡེ་ཤེས་སྐར་ཁུང་ནི། སྐྱིལ་ཀྲུང་བྱ་
ལ་ལག་སོར་བཞི་ཕོ་བ་ལ་སྦྱར། མཐེ་བོང་གཉིས་ཀྱིས་
དཔྱི་མགོ་གཡས་གཡོན་བཟུང་། གྲུ་མོའི་ཁུག་ཏུ་གྲུ་གསུམ་
སྐར་ཁུང་དོང་པར་བྱས་ཏེ། པུས་མོ་གཡས་གཡོན་སྟེང་དུ་
བཞག་ལ། ཕྱིར་བསྒྲིལ་སྤྱི་བོ་ས་ལ་བཙུག་པ། ནང་བསྒྲིལ་
དཔྲལ་བ་ས་ལ་བཙུག་པ་ལན་བདུན་བྱ།

6. Striking the Athlete's Hammer to Overcome Hatred

Hold the nape of your neck with the interlaced fingers of your two hands. Plant your two knees on the ground with the back of your two ankles interlaced behind you. Load your weight on the knees, straighten your waist, and then bend downward so that your two elbows touch your two knees. Do this seven times.

7. The Skylight of Primordial Wisdom to Overcome Delusion

Sitting cross-legged, place the four fingers of each hand on your stomach. Your two thumbs hold the left and right hip bones. Bend your elbows to form a triangular skylight; place your elbows on top of your right and left knees. Roll backward planting your crown on the ground. Roll forward planting your forehead on the ground. Do this seven times.

བརྒྱད་པ་ང་རྒྱལ་འཁོར་ལོ་བཞི་བསྒྲིལ་ནི། སེམས་དཔའི་སྐྱིལ་ཀྲུང་བྱ་ལ་བརྣ་གཡས་གཡོན་འོག་ཏུ་རྐང་མགོ་གཉིས་མནན། ཚང་པ་གཉིས་ཀྱིས་རྐང་པའི་མཐེ་བོང་གཡས་གཡོན་བཟུང་ལ། ཕྱི་རུ་བསྒྲིལ་ནས་ལྟག་པ་ས་ལ་བཙུག །ནང་དུ་བསྒྲིལ་[328]ནས་པུས་མོ་བཙུག་སྐྱིད་ཁུག་རྐེད་པ་ཤད་ཀྱིས་བསྲང་། དེ་ལྟར་ཕྱིར་བསྒྲིལ་ནང་བསྒྲིལ་ལན་བདུན་བྱ།

དགུ་པ་འདོད་ཆགས་རྒྱ་མདུད་ཟུར་བཀྲོལ་ནི། སེམས་དཔའི་སྐྱིལ་ཀྲུང་བཅའ་ལ་གྲུ་མོ་གཉིས་བརྒྱང་། མཐེ་བོང་གཉིས་ཀྱིས་མཆན་ཁུང་གཡས་གཡོན་མནན། སོར་མོ་བཞི་པོའི་རྩེ་མོ་ཐུགས་ཀར་སྦྲད། གྲུ་མོ་གཡས་པས་པུས་མོ་གཡོན་ལ་ཐུག་པ་དང་། གཡོན་གྱིས་གཡས་ལ་ཐུག་པ་སྟེ། གཡས་གཙུས་གཡོན་གཙུས་ལན་བདུན་བྱ།

8. Rolling the Four Limbs like Wheels to Overcome Pride

Sitting in the bodhisattva cross-legged posture, press the top of each foot beneath the right and left thighs. Your two hands hold the left and right big toes. Rolling backward plant the nape of your neck on the ground. Rolling forward plant your knees. At the bend of the knee straighten your waist. In this way, roll backward and forward seven times.

9. Loosening the Corner of the Braided Knot to Overcome Attachment

Assuming the bodhisattva cross-legged posture, extend both elbows. With each thumb press under your corresponding right and left armpits. The tips of the four fingers meet at the heart. The right elbow touches the left knee and the left touches the right. In this way twist to the right and twist to the left seven times, alternating.

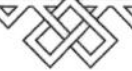

བཅུ་པ་ཕྲག་དོག་དར་ལྕེ་གྲེན་སྦྱུགས་ནི། རྐང་གཡོན་བྲང་ང་དང་ལག་གཡོན་པའི་མཐིལ་གཉིས་ས་ལ་བཙུག །རྐང་ལག་གཡས་གཉིས་གནམ་དུ་སྦྱུགས་བརྒྱང་ལན་བདུན་བྱ། ཡང་རྐང་ལག་གཡས་གཉིས་ས་ལ་བཙུག །གཡོན་གཉིས་གནམ་དུ་སྦྱུགས་བརྐྱང་[329]ལན་བདུན་བྱ། བཅུ་གཅིག་པ་བྱིང་རྒོད་སྟག་མོ་མཆོངས་སྟབས་ནི། ལག་པ་གཉིས་རྐང་པའི་སྨྱིད་ཁུག་ཕྱི་ནས་ནང་དུ་དྲངས་ལ་རྣ་བ་གཉིས་ལ་འཇུས་ཤིང་མགོ་བོ་བཀུག་རྐང་མཐིལ་གཉིས་ས་ལ་བཙུག་ལ་མདུན་དུ་ལན་བདུན་མཆོངས། ཕྱི་ལའང་དེ་ལྟར་བདུན་མཆོངས། ཀུན་ལ་གསིགས་སྦྱུགས་ཧ་ཕཊ༔ སྒྲ་འདོན་འགྲེས་སོ། །ཚ་བའི་འཁྲུལ་འཁོར་ལྔ་པོ་འདི་དཔོན་རྒྱལ་བཙན་པོའི་དགོངས་པའོ།

10. Waving the Silk Tassel Upward to Overcome Jealousy

Plant the edge of the left foot and palm of the left hand on the ground. Extend both the right leg and arm, waving them to the sky seven times. Also, then plant both the right foot and hand on the ground. Extend the two, the left arm and leg, waving them to the sky seven times.

11. The Stance of a Tigress's Leap to Overcome Drowsiness and Agitation

Bring the two hands from the outside of the knee-joints to the inside. Bend the head and hold the two ears. With soles of both feet planted on the ground, jump forward seven times. Then also jump backward seven times in the same manner.

In all magical movements shake and shudder while sounding *ha* and *phat*.

These five root magical movements are the exalted perspective of Pongyal Tsenpo.

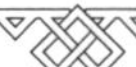

།འདི་ལྷའི་ཡོན་ཏན་ནི། སྙན་བརྒྱུད་ཞལ་ཤེས་ལས་བཏུས་པ། དུག་ལྔའི་རྩ་སྒོ་འགག་ཅིང་ཡེ་ཤེས་རྩ་སྒོ་འབྱེད། ཕུང་ལྔ་གནས་སུ་དག་ཅིང་སྐུ་ལྔའི་དཀྱིལ་འཁོར་རྫོགས། འབྱུང་ལྔ་དབང་དུ་འདུས་ཤིང་དྭངས་མ་འོད་ལྔ་འཆར། ཞེས་དང་། བྱིང་རྒོད་སྡུག་མོ་མཆོངས་སྟབས་ཡོན་ཏན་ནི། སྲོག་རླུང་ཤུགས་རྣམས་རྫོགས་[330]ཅིང་བྱིང་རྒོད་རང་སར་སངས། རླུང་སེམས་དབུ་མར་ཚུད་ཅིང་རྟོག་ཚོགས་འགྱུ་བྱེད་གྲོལ། ཞེས་སོ།

Benefits

As for the benefits of these five, as summarized from *Quintessential Oral Insructions*: "The door to the channel of the five poisons is closed, and the door to the channel of primordial wisdom is opened. The five aggregates are purified in their own place, and the mandala of the five enlightened bodies is perfected. The five elements are controlled and the five radiant lights arise." The benefit of the "stance of the tigress's leap" is that the power of the life-holding wind is perfected, and drowsiness and agitation are naturally purified. Wind and mind enter into the central channel and the rush of the hordes of thoughts are liberated.

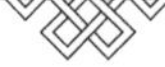

༄༅ གེགས་སེལ་དྲུག་ནི། ངང་མོ་ཆུ་འཐུང་། འཁྲོང་མོ་ཟུར་བརྡུང་། རྐྱང་མོའི་ཉལ་སྟབས། ཁྲ་ཡི་ཀླུང་འཛིན། གླིང་བཞི་མཐའ་བསྒྲིལ། གླིང་བཞི་མཐའ་རྒྱས་སོ། །བཅུ་གཉིས་པ་ངང་མོ་ཆུ་འཐུང་ནི། ལུས་པོ་བསྲང་ལ་རྐེད་པ་ཆང་པས་བཟུང་ལ་མཐེ་བོང་གཉིས་ནང་དུ་བསྣན། ནང་དུ་རྒྱུར་ནས་སྤྱི་བོས་ས་ལ་རེག་པ་དང་། ཤད་ཀྱིས་ལངས་ལ་མགོ་བོ་ལྟག་པར་དཀྱེད། དེ་ལྟར་ཕྱིར་དཀྱེད་ནང་རྒྱུར་རེས་མོ་ལན་བདུན་བྱ། གསིགས་སྦྱུགས་དང་ཧ་པཊཿའགྲེས།

Root Magical Movement Set that Clears Away Obstacles

The six root magical movements that clear away obstacles are "duck drinking water," "wild yak butting sideways," "female donkey lying down to sleep," "kestrel hovering in the wind," "rolling up the limits of the four continents," and "extending the limits of the four continents."

12. Duck Drinking Water

Straighten the standing body and hold the waist with the hands, the two thumbs pointing forward. Bow forward touching the crown toward the ground and then rise like a brushstroke and bend the head backward at the neck. In that way bend backward and bow forward seven times. Shake and stir, and apply the *ha phat*.

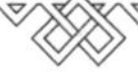

བཅུ་གསུམ་པ་འཁྲོང་མོ་ཟུར་བརྡུང་ནི། ལངས་ལ་མཇུབ་མོ་ནང་དུ་བསྟན་ནས་རྐེད་པར་བཟུང་། རོ་སྟོད་དཔུང་མགོ་པུས་མོ་གཡས་ལ་བཀལ་ནས་[331]གཡས་ཟུར་ནས་མགོ་བོས་བརྡུང་ཚུལ་བྱེད་ཅིང་། རྐང་པ་བསྒོལ་མར་མཆོངས་སྟབས་སུ་གཡོན་ལའང་དེ་དང་འདྲ་སྟེ། རེས་མོས་དཀྲུས་མཆོངས་ལན་བདུན་བྱ། བཅུ་བཞི་རྐྱང་མོའི་ཉལ་སྟབས་ནི། ལུས་པོ་ལངས་ལ་མཇུབ་མོ་ནང་དུ་བསྟན་ནས་རྐེད་པར་བཟུང་། རོ་སྟོད་བསྒྱུར་ལ་གྲུ་མོ་གཡས་པས་པུས་མོ་གཡོན་དང་། གཡོན་པས་གཡས་ལ་རེག་ཙམ་བྱ་ཞིང་། རྐང་པ་ཕྱེད་བསྣལ་གཡས་གཡོན་བསྒོལ་མར་སྟོད་སྨད་དཀྲུས་ལ་ལན་བདུན་བྱ།

13. Wild Yak Butting Sideways

Standing, with your fingers pointing to the front, hold the waist. Lean the torso, the shoulder, and head toward the right knee, angle to the right, then the head makes a butting motion and cross the legs with a hop. Perform similarly to the left. Alternate this twisting and jumping seven times.

14. Female Donkey Lying Down to Sleep

Standing, with your fingers pointing to the front, hold the waist. Turning your torso, touch the left knee with the right elbow, and then touch the right knee with the left elbow. Halfway lie down the legs each time. Alternating right and left, twist the upper torso and the lower legs seven times.

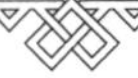

བཅོ་ལྔ་པ་ཁྲ་ཡི་རླུང་འཛིན་ནི། རྐང་པ་གཉིས་གཤིབས་ནས་ལངས་ལ་ཆང་པས་རྐེད་པར་བཟུང་ལ་མཐེ་བོང་ནང་དུ་བསྣུན། རྐང་མཐིལ་ཙུང་ཙམ་བརྟེགས་ལ་མགོ་དང་རོ་སྟོད་གཡས་བསྒྱུར་གཡོན་བསྒྱུར་རྒྱབ་བསྒྱུར་རེ་དང་། གནམ་ལ་འཕག་པ་རེ་བྱ་བ་དེ་འདྲ་[332]ལན་བདུན་བྱ། བཅུ་དྲུག་པ་གླིང་བཞི་མཐའ་བསྒྲིལ་ནི། ལངས་ལ་རྐང་པ་གཡས་ཀྱིས་གཡོན་པའི་བྲུས་གོང་དུ་རེག་ཙམ་རེ་བྱ་ཞིང་གཡོན་ཡང་འདྲ་ལ། ལག་པ་གཡས་གཡོན་མཆན་ཁུང་དུ་བསྣོལ་མར་བསྒྲིལ་བ་ལན་བདུན་བྱ།

15. Kestrel Hovering in the Wind

Stand with both feet together. Then, hold your waist with your hands, your thumbs pointing forward. Slightly lift the soles of the feet and turn the head and torso to the right, to the left and to the back, rising upward to the sky each time. Do this seven times.

16. Rolling Up the Limits of the Four Continents

While standing, touch your left leg above the knee with your right leg, and then touch the right leg with the left. Simultaneously, with the right hand touch the left armpit and and with the left hand touch the right armpit. Alternate circling seven times.

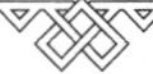

བཅུ་བདུན་པ་གླིང་བཞི་མཐའ་རྒྱས་ནི། རྡོ་རྗེ་སྐྱིལ་ཀྲུང་བཅའ་ལ་ལག་པ་གཉིས་ཀྱི་སྲིན་ལག་གིས་མཐེ་བོང་མནན་ཏེ་ལག་མགོ་ས་ལ་བཙུག །ལྷེད་རྣམས་ལག་པར་བཀལ་ནས་ལུས་པོ་ཡར་ལ་བཏེགས་ཤིང་འབེབ་བསྐོར་བདུན་བྱའོ། །འདི་དག་གི་ཡོན་ཏན་ནི། ཞལ་ཤེས་ནས། ངང་མོས་བཞི་བསྡུས་ནད་ལས་གྲོལ་ཞིང་ནམ་མཁའི་རྩ་སྒོ་འབྱེད།། འབྲིང་མོས་བད་ཀན་ནད་ལས་གྲོལ་ཞིང་ས་ཡི་རྩ་སྒོ་འབྱེད།། རྐྱང་མོས་མཁྲིས་པའི་ནད་ལས་གྲོལ་ཞིང་རླུང་གི་རྩ་སྒོ་འབྱེད། ཁྲ་ཡིས་ཚ་བའི་ནད་[333]ལས་གྲོལ་ཞིང་མེ་མི་རྩ་སྒོ་འབྱེད། གླིང་བཞིས་གྲང་བའི་ནད་ལས་གྲོལ་ཞིང་ཆུ་ཡི་རྩ་སྒོ་འབྱེད། ཐུན་མོང་བང་མགྱོགས་སྟོབས་ལྡན་དྲོད་འབར་ཚེ་རིང་ལོག་པོར་འགྱུར། རྟོག་མེད་ཞིག་པོས་གསུངས་པའོ། །ཞེས་སོ།

17. Extending the Limits of the Four Continents

Assuming the *vajra* cross-legged posture, press the thumbs with the base of the ring finger of each hand into a fist, and plant the top of the fist on the ground. Having loaded all your weight on your hands, raise the body up and drop it while rotating. Do this seven times.

Benefits

The benefits of these, according to *Quintessential Oral Instructions*, are the following:

> The "duck" liberates from the diseases of the four consituents (phlegm, bile, wind, and the combination of the three) and opens the door of the channel of the space element; the "wild yak" liberates from the diseases of phlegm and opens the door of the channel of the earth element; the "female donkey" liberates from diseases of bile and opens the door of the channel of the air element; the "kestrel" liberates from diseases of heat and opens the door of the channel of fire; and the "four continents" liberates from diseases of cold and opens the door of the channel of water. The common benefits of these magical movements are speed-walking, power, blazing warmth, and reversing the aging process. This has been stated by Togme Shigpo.

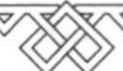

༄ ཡན་ལག་གི་འཁྲུལ་འཁོར་ལ། རྩ་བ་ལྔ། གེགས་སེལ་
ལྔའོ། །རྩ་བ་ལྔ་ནི། འབྱུང་བཞི་རང་འབེབ། རྨ་བྱ་ཆུ་འཐུང་།
སྟོང་པ་བཞི་འདུས། སྟེང་འོག་བཞི་བསྐྱིལ། རྒྱ་མདུད་བཞི་
རྡེག་གོ །བཅོ་བརྒྱད་པ་འབྱུང་བཞི་རང་འབེབ་ནི། སྐྱིལ་
ཀྲུང་འདུག་ལ་ལག་མཐིལ་གཉིས་ཀྱིས་བརླ་ལ་མནན་ཅིང་
ལུས་དང་ལག་ངར་བསྲང་། མགོ་དང་རོ་སྟོད་ནང་དུ་
སྒྱུགས་པ་ཕྱི་ཙུ་དབྱེ་བ་དེ་འདྲ་ལན་བདུན་བྱ།

Branch Magical Movement Cycle

The branch magical movements are also composed of five root movements and five that clear away obstacles.

Root Branch Movements

The five root branch movements are "natural descent of the four elements," "peacock drinking water," "collecting the four stalks," "rolling the four upper and lower limbs," and "striking the four braided knots."

18. Natural Descent of the Four Elements

Sitting in the cross-legged position, press your two palms on the thighs and straighten the body and arms. Shake the head and torso leaning forward and then leaning back up. Do this seven times.

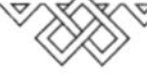

བཅུ་དགུ་པ་རྨ་བྱ་ཆུ་འཐུང་ནི། རྐང་པ་གཉིས་གཞིབས་
ལ་མདུན་དུ་བརྐྱང་། [334]ལག་ངར་རྒྱབ་ཏུ་བསྣོལ་ལ་
སྲིན་མཛུབ་མཐེ་བོང་གིས་མནན། ལུས་པོ་ནང་དུ་བཀུག་
ལ་དཔྲལ་བ་པུས་མོའི་བར་དུ་རེག་ཙམ་རེ་དང་། མགོ་བོ་
གྱེན་དུ་བཏེགས་ཞིང་འཕྲུག་གོང་དུ་གཡས་བལྟ་གཡོན་
བལྟ་རེ་དང་། གནམ་དུ་བལྟ་བ་རེ་དང་གསུམ་རེ་བྱ་བ།
དེ་ལྟར་ལན་བདུན་བྱ།

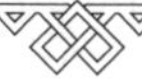

19. Peacock Drinking Water

With your two legs aligned, extend them in front. Join or cross your arms behind your back, thumbs pressing the base of the ring fingers. Bend your body forward until your forehead touches the knees. Then raise your head and look to the right above your shoulder and look to the left above your shoulder, and look to the sky. Perform each of these three (i.e., right, left and to the sky). Do this seven times.

ཉི་ཤུ་པ་སྡོང་པོ་བཞི་འདུས་ནི། འདུག་ལ་རྐང་པའི་མཐེ་བོང་གཡས་གཡོན་ཆང་པ་གཉིས་ཀྱིས་བཟུང་ནས་སྐལ་ཚོགས་ས་ལ་བཙུག་ཅིང་། རྐང་ལག་བཞི་གནམ་དུ་བརྐྱང་ཞིང་གྱེས་རྩལ་བྱ་བ་དེ་འདྲ་ལན་བདུན་བྱ། ཉེར་གཅིག་པ་སྟེང་འོག་བཞི་བསྒྲིལ་ནི། རྐང་མགོ་གཡས་གཡོན་ཆང་པ་གཉིས་ཀྱིས་བཟུང་ལ། ཕྱི་རུ་བསྒྲིལ་ནས་རྐང་མགོ་ས་ལ་བཙུག་ནང་དུ་བསྒྲིལ་ནས་དཔྲལ་བ་ས་ལ་བཙུག །དེ་བཞིན་ལན་བདུན་བྱ།

20. Collecting the Four Stalks

Seated, holding your right and left big toes with your two hands, plant your spine on the ground. Extend the four—two arms and two legs—to the sky and spread them out. Do this seven times.

21. Rolling the Four Upper and Lower Limbs

Sitting cross legged, hold the top of your left and right feet with your two hands, roll backward, planting the top of your feet on the ground, then roll forward, planting the forehead on the ground. Repeat like this seven times.

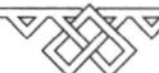

ཉེར་གཉིས་པ་རྒྱ་[335]མདུད་བཞི་རྡེག་ནི། རྡོ་རྗེ་སྐྱིལ་ཀྲུང་བྱ་ལ་སྒྲིད་ཁུག་བར་ནས་ལག་པ་གཡས་གཡོན་བརྡོན་ཏེ། ཆང་པ་གཉིས་ཀྱིས་བྱིན་པའི་འོག་ནས་ཡར་བཟུང་ལ་འབེབ་བསྐོར་ལན་བདུན་བྱའོ། །གཟུགས་བཞི་གསེགས་སྐྱུགས་ཧ་ཕཊ༔ སྦྲ་འདོན་ཀུན་ལ་དགོས། འདི་དག་གི་ཡོན་ཏན་ནི། སྙན་བརྒྱུད་ཞལ་ཤེས་ལས། འབྱུང་བཞིའི་ནད་ལས་གྲོལ་ཞིང་རླུང་སེམས་གནད་དུ་ཚུད།། སྣང་བ་སྒྱུ་མར་གྲོལ་ཅིང་འཁྲུལ་སྣང་ཞེན་པ་ལྡོག །ལུས་ཀྱི་སྟོབས་རྒྱས་འབྱུང་བཞི་རང་དབང་ཐོབ། ཕྱི་ནང་གེགས་རྣམས་སེལ་ཅིང་རྩ་རླུང་གནད་དུ་ཚུད། ལུས་སྒྱུམ་དྲོད་འབར་མདངས་ལེགས་སྟོབས་རྣམས་རྒྱས། ཞེས་སོ།

22. Striking the Four Braided Knots

Sitting in the *vajra* cross-legged posture, put the right and left hands into the kneepits. Your two hands hold up the calfs from below. Raise the body up, turn, and drop it seven times. Shuddering and shaking the four limbs, then reciting the sounds *ha phat* are required for all movements.

Benefits

As for the benefits, *Quintessential Oral Instructions from the Aural Transmission of Zhang Zhung* states:

> The benefits are as follows: Liberation from the diseases of the four elements. Wind and mind penetrate the vital points making the body function well. Appearances are liberated as illusions, and attachment to deluded appearances is reversed. The strength of the body is increased. You obtain natural mastery over the four elements. External and internal obstacles are cleared, and the winds penetrate the vital points of the channels making the body function well. The oily blazing-warmth of the body blazes radiantly. The excellent strength of the body is increased.

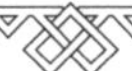

༄ གེགས་སེལ་ལྔ་ནི། ཁྲུང་ཆེན་གཞོག་རྡེབ། རྨ་བྱ་ཆུ་སྐྱུགས། བཞི་འདུས་[336]མཐའ་སེལ། ཨེ་ནའི་ཟུར་འགྲོས། ཤ་རའི་ཟུར་སྐྱུགས་སོ། །ཉེར་གསུམ་པ་ཁྲུང་ཆེན་གཞོག་རྡེབ་ནི། ཤད་ཀྱིས་ལངས་ལ་ལག་གཡས་སྤྱི་བོའི་ནམ་མཁའ་ལ་བརྐྱང་པ་དང་། རྐང་པ་གཡས་པའི་ཕྱི་རྟིང་འཕོངས་ཞབས་སུ་རེག་པ་དུས་མཉམ་དུ་བྱ། ལག་པ་གཡོན་དཔྱི་ཐད་ནས་ཕྱུར་དུ་བརྐྱང་། དེ་ལྟར་གཡས་གཡོན་རེས་མོ་ལན་བདུན་བྱ།

The Branch Magical Movement Set that Clear Away Obstacles

The five branch magical movements that clear away obstacles are "great garuda flapping its wings," "peacock shaking off water," "collecting the four limbs, clearing away the limitations," "antelope galloping sideways," and "deer shaking sideways."

23. Great Garuda Flapping Its Wings

Standing upright, extend the right arm to the apex of the sky and simultaneously touch the right heel to your buttocks. Extend the left hand from the hip downward. Repeat, alternating left and right seven times.

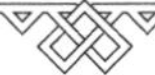

ཉེར་བཞི་པ་རྨ་བྱ་ཆུ་སྤྱུགས་ནི། ལངས་ལ་ལག་པ་གཉིས་
མདུན་དུ་གཞིབས་ནས་ལག་མཐིལ་ས་ལ་བསྟན་ཏེ།
མདུན་དང་གཡས་གཡོན་གསུམ་ལ་ལག་མགོ་གཉིས་
དུས་གཅིག་ཏུ་སྤྱུགས་པ་ལན་བདུན་བྱ། ཉེར་ལྔ་པ་བཞི་
འདུས་མཐའ་སེལ་ནི། རྐང་མཐིལ་གཉིས་སྦྱར་ནས་འདུག་
ལ་ལག་པ་གཉིས་ཀྱིས་རྐང་མགོ་ལ་བཟུང་སྟེ། མདུན་དུ་
ལན་བདུན་[337]མཆོངས། རྒྱབ་ཏུ་ཕྱི་ལ་བདུན་མཆོངས།

24. Peacock Shaking Off Water

Standing, with both arms parallel in front, palms facing the ground, simultaneously shake the tops of both hands to three directions: front, right, and left. Do this seven times.

25. Collecting the Four Limbs, Clearing Away Limitations

Sitting with the soles of the two feet together, hold the top of the feet with both hands. Then, jump forward seven times and jump backward seven times.

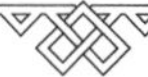

ཉེར་དྲུག་པ་ཨེ་ནའི་བྲུར་འགྲོས་ནི། རྐང་མགོ་གཡོན་པ་
ལག་པ་གཡོན་པས་བཟུང་ལ་རྐང་མཐིལ་རྒྱུ་ཞབས་གཡས་
སུ་སྦྱར། རྐང་པ་གཡས་པ་མཆོངས་འགྲོས་བྱ་ཞིང་།
ལག་གཡས་དཔྱི་ཐད་ནས་སྒྱུགས་པ་དུས་མཉམ་པ། དེ་
འདྲ་མདུན་དུ་མཆོངས་ཚུང་བདུན། རྒྱབ་ཏུ་ཁ་ཕྱི་ལ་
འཁོར་ནས་བདུན་བྱ། གཡོན་ཡང་དེ་དང་འདྲ་བ་བརྗེ་
ལན་བྱ།

26. Antelope Galloping Sideways

Holding the top of the left foot with the left hand, place the sole of that foot at the bottom-right side of the intestines. Hop forward on the right foot while shaking the right hand from the hip. In this manner, take seven small hops forward. Having turned around, take seven small hops back. Shifting your weight, do this similarly on the left.

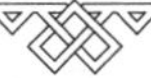

ཉེར་བདུན་པ་ཤ་རའི་བྲུར་སྦྲུགས་ནི། ལངས་ལ་རྐང་མཐིལ་གཡས་པས་ཐེར་ཁྱུག་མནན། ལག་པ་གཉིས་ཐུར་སེལ་བྲུར་ནས་བརྐྱང་། རོ་སྟོད་དཔུང་མགོ་བཀུག་ལ་རྐང་གཡོན་མཆོངས་ཆུང་རེ་དང་རོ་སྟོད་ཀྱུར་ཚུལ་གསུམ་རེ་སྤྲད་པ་མདུན་དུ་བདུན་རྒྱབ་ཏུ་ཕྱི་ལ་འཁོར་ནས་བདུན་བྱ། [338]གཡོན་ཡང་དེ་དང་འདྲ་བ་བརྗེ་ལན་རླུང་ཁྱུག་གཅིག་ལ་བྱའོ།

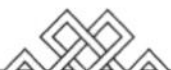

27. Deer Shaking Sideways

Standing, press the sole of the right foot against the hollow spot of the left leg. Extend both hands from the side in a downward, clearing manner. Bending the torso, shoulders, and head, make a small hop with the left leg, and with each hop bend your torso forward three times, hopping seven times in all. Then, turn around and do this seven times to the back. Do this similarly to the left. Do this all in one cycle of breath.

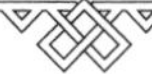

།འདི་དག་གི་ཡོན་ཏན་ནི། སྔ་མ་ལས། འབྱུང་བའི་གེགས་གྲོལ་འབྱུང་བཞིའི་རྩ་སྒོ་འབྱེད།། འབྱུང་བ་ཆ་སྙོམས་བཞི་བསྐྱུས་ནད་མི་ཚུགས། ཡན་ལག་གི་འཁྲུལ་འཁོར་བཅུ་པོ་འདི་དག་ལྷུན་གྲུབ་སྨུ་ཕྱུར་གྱི་དགོངས་པའོ། ༔ བྱེ་བྲག་གི་འཁྲུལ་འཁོར་ལ། མགོ་ལུས་ཡན་ལག་སོ་སོའི་གེགས་སེལ་དང་། ཐུན་མོང་གི་གེགས་སེལ་ལོ། མགོ་དང་། རོ་སྟོད་དང་། ལག་པ་དང་། རྐེད་པ་དང་། རྐང་པའི་གེགས་སེལ་ལྔའོ།

Benefits

As for the benefits of these, from the former (i.e., *Quintessential Oral Instructions*):

> The obstacles from the elements are liberated. The doors to the channels of the elements are opened. The elements are balanced. You are unharmed by the collection of the four diseases.

These ten branch magical movements (five root and five that clear obstacles) are in accordance with the perspective of Lhundrub Muthur.

Distinctive Magical Movement Set that Clears Away Specific Obstacles

As for the distinctive magical movements, there are the movements that clear the obstacles of each of the head, body, and limbs individually, and there are the movements that clear away the obstacles that are in common among the head and so forth.

There are five magical movements that clear away the specific obstacles of the head, torso, arms, waist, and legs.

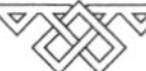

།ཉེར་བརྒྱད་པ་མགོའི་གེགས་སེལ་མགོ་རིལ་མགོ་ཀྱོག་ནི། སྐྱིལ་ཀྲུང་བྱ་ལ་ལག་གཉིས་བརླ་སྟེང་བསྒྲེངས། མགོ་བོ་གཡས་གཡོན་དུ་བདུན་རེ་བསྐོར་ཞིང་མདུན་རྒྱབ་ཏུ་བཀུག་དབྱེད་ལན་བདུན་བྱ། [339]ཉེར་དགུ་པ་རོ་སྟོད་ཀྱི་ཤིང་སྒྲོགས་ཆེངས་ནི། འདུག་ལ་ལག་གཉིས་སྙིང་ཁར་བསྣོལ་ཏེ་འཕྲུག་མགོ་གཡས་གཡོན་བཟུང་། ཕུས་མོ་གཉིས་ས་ལ་བཙུག་ནས། རོ་སྟོད་གཙུས་ཞིང་གཡས་སུ་བདུན་གཡོན་དུ་བདུན་བསྐོར་བར་བྱ།

28. Clearing Obstacles from the Head: Rotating and Nodding the Head

Sitting cross-legged, extend both hands on top of the thighs. Rotate the head to the right and left seven times each, and then bend to the front and back seven times.

29. Swinging the Binding Chains of the Torso

Sitting with both arms crossed at the heart, hold the shoulders to the right and left sides of the head. After planting both knees on the ground, twist the torso and rotate seven times to the right and seven to the left.

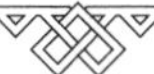

སུམ་ཅུ་པ་ལག་པ་ཕོ་རོག་སྤྱེར་འཛིན་ནི། སེམས་དཔའི་
སྐྱིལ་ཀྲུང་འདུག་ལ་ལག་པ་གཉིས་ཀྱི་སྐྲར་མོ་གཟེངས་ལ་
གཡས་གཡོན་རེག་མོས་བརྒྱང་བརྐྱུམ་སོར་བཀྲོལ་བདུན་
བདུན་བྱ། སོ་གཅིག་པ་ཕོ་བ་རྡོ་རྗེ་རང་འཁོར་ནི། སེམས་
དཔའི་སྐྱིལ་ཀྲུང་བཅའ་ལ་གྲུ་མོ་གཡས་གཡོན་བསྐྱོལ་བར་
ཚང་པས་བཟུང་། ལག་ངར་བརྩེགས་ནས་རྐེད་པ་བསྐྱོམ་
ལ་ཕོ་བ་གཡས་སུ་བདུན་གཡོན་དུ་བདུན་བསྐོར་བར་བྱ།

30. Grasping with the Raven's Claws, Clearing Away the Obstacles of the Arms

Sitting in the bodhisattva posture, flex the palms of both hands, alternating between the right and left, extending out and drawing in, releasing the fingers. Do this seven times for each hand.

31. *Vajra* Self-Rotation of the Stomach

Assuming the cross-legged bodhisattva posture, crossing the right and left elbows hold the stomach with the hands. Having folded stacked the forearms on top of each other, clasp the waist and rotate the stomach seven times to the right and seven times to the left.

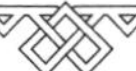

སོ་གཉིས་པ་རྐང་པ་ཛ་མོང་འདོར་སྟབས་ནི། ཚོག་ཕུར་འདུག་ལ་ལག་ངར་རྐང་པའི་བར་[340]ནས་བཏོན་ལ་རྐང་པའི་མཐེ་བོང་ལག་པ་གཉིས་ཀྱིས་བཟུང་། རྒྱབ་ཏུ་བསྒྲིལ་ནས་རྐང་མགོ་ས་ལ་བཙུག །རྐང་ལག་ཤེད་ཀྱིས་སྒྲུགས་ལ་བརྐྱང་། དེ་འདྲ་ལན་བདུན་བྱའོ། །གཟུགས་བཞི་སྒྲུགས་ཤིང་ཧ་ཕཊ༔སོགས་ཀུན་ལ་འདྲེས། འདི་དག་གི་ཡོན་ཏན་ནི། ཚ་གྲང་རླུང་མཁྲིས་གདོན་རྐྱེན་ཐམས་ཅད་སེལ། ཡན་ལག་སོ་སོའི་ནད་རྣམས་སེལ་བར་འགྱུར། འོར་སྒོམ་ཀུན་འདུལ་གྱི་དགོངས་པའོ།

32. Camel's Fighting Stance that Clears Away the Obstacles of the Legs

Sitting on the floor, extend the forearms between the legs, and hold the big toes with both hands. Rolling backward, plant the top of the foot on the ground. Then shake and extend with the legs and arms straight like a brush-stroke. Do this seven times. Shake the four limbs and sound *ha* and *phat*. Integrate these with all other movements.

Benefits

As for the benefits, the perspective of Orgom Kundul is that all the cooperative conditions of heat, cold, wind, bile, and demons are cleared. Also, the diseases of each of the limbs are cleared.

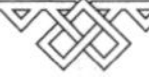

༄ །ཐུན་མོང་གེགས་སེལ་ལ། རྒྱ་མཚོ་གཏིང་སྤྲུགས། རྒྱ་
མདུད་དགུ་བཀྲོལ། རྩ་འདུལ་རྩ་བཀྲོལ། རྒྱ་མོ་དར་ཐག
དང་པོ། གཉིས་པ། གསུམ་པ། ནོར་བུ་འཕར་ལེན་ནོ། སོ་
གསུམ་པ་རྒྱ་མཚོ་གཏིང་སྤྲུགས་ནི། སེམས་དཔའི་སྐྱིལ་
ཀྲུང་བཅའ་ལ་ལག་ངར་ཕྱིར་བསྟན། སོར་མོ་གཉིས་ཀྱིས་
[341]རྐང་ངར་འོག་ནས་ཡར་བཟུང་ལ་གཡས་བདུན་
གཡོན་བདུན་བསྐོར། དེ་ནས་རྐང་ངར་རྐེད་པ་ཤད་ཀྱིས་
བསྲང་ལ་ལུས་པོ་ཀུན་སྤྲུགས་པ་ཅི་མང་བྱ།

DISTINCTIVE MAGICAL MOVEMENT SET THAT CLEARS AWAY COMMON OBSTACLES

The magical movements that clear away common obstacles are "shaking the depths of the ocean," "loosening the nine braided knots," "disciplining and loosening the channels," "Chinese woman weaving silk" (parts one, two, and three), and "bouncing jewel."

33. SHAKING THE DEPTHS OF THE OCEAN

Assuming the bodhisattva posture, point your arms out. Holding your calves from underneath with your four fingers of each hand, rotate seven times to the right and seven times to the left. Then, straightening the legs and waist like a brushstroke, shake your whole body as many times as possible.

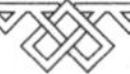

སོ་བཞི་པ་རྒྱ་མདུད་དགུ་བཀྲོལ་ནི། འདུག་ལ་རྐང་པ་གཉིས་ཕྱེད་བརྐྱང་ཙམ་བྱ། ལག་མཐིལ་གཉིས་ཀྱིས་རེས་མོས་སྒྲི་བོ། །དཔྲལ་བ། ལྟག་ཁུང་། འཕྲག་མགོ་གཡས་གཡོན། དཔྱི་མིག་གཡས་གཡོན། ཕྱུས་མགོ་གཡས་གཡོན་ལ་བདུན་རེ་བརྡེག་ཅིང་། རྐང་པའི་རྟིང་པ་ས་ལ་བརྡེག་དེ་ནས་ལག་མཐིལ་གཉིས་ས་ལ་བཙུག་ལ། རོ་སྨད་གནམ་ལ་ལན་གསུམ་འཕང་སྟེ་རྐང་མཐིལ་ས་ལ་བརྡབ། དེ་ནས་ཤད་ཀྱིས་ལངས་ལ་འཕེབ་ཆེན་གསུམ་རྒྱབ་ལ། བར་སྣང་ལ་སེམས་དཔའི་སྐྱིལ་ཀྲུང་བྱ་ལ་འདུག་པ་གསུམ་མཆན། གསིགས་སྤྲུགས་སོགས་འདྲ།

34. Loosening the Nine Braided Knots

Sitting with both legs half bent, tap with both palms seven times each: the crown of the head, the forehead, the base of the nape of the neck, the top of the right and left shoulders, the right and left hip bones, the top of the right and left knees. Stomp the ground with the heels. Then plant the palms of both hands on the ground, throw the lower part of your body into the air three times; then let the soles of the feet fall to the ground. Following that, stand upright striking three times the great descent and return to the ground on your buttocks. (While in the air, sit in the *bodhisattva* cross-legged posture three times.) Shudder, shake, and so forth, similar to other movements.

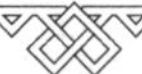

[342]སོ་ལྷ་པ་རྩ་འདུལ་རྩ་བཀྲོལ་ནི། ལངས་ལ་མཐེ་བོང་ནང་དུ་བསྣུན་ནས་ཆང་པ་གཉིས་ཀྱིས་རྐེད་པར་བཟུང་། རྩ་གསུམ་འཁོར་ལོ་དྲུག་ཐབས་ཤེས་ཀྱི་ཡིག་ལི་རྣམས་གསལ་གདབ་ལ། སྤྱི་བོའི་རྩ་འཁོར་ཨཿ མགྲིན་པར་ཨོཾ་ ཐུགས་ཀར་ཧཱུྃཿ རྐང་མཐིལ་འཁོར་ལོ་ཡཾ། གསང་བར་རཾ། ལྟེ་བར་ཁཾ། དེ་ནས་གཏུམ་མོ་མེས་རྩ་ཁམས་དྲོས་ནས་ཨཿ ཨོཾ་ ཧཱུྃཿ གསུམ་འོད་དུ་ཞུ་སྟེ། ཡིག་ལི་དཀར་དམར་མཐིང་གསུམ་དུ་གྱུར་ནས་རྐང་མཐིལ་ཡཾཿ ལ་ཐིམ། ཡཾ་ལས་རླུང་གཡོས། རཾ་ལས་མེ་འབར། ཁཾ་ལས་བདུད་རྩི་བབས། དེ་ལས་རླུང་མེ་འོད་སེར་པོའི་རྣམ་པ་བྱུང་ནས་དུས་གསུམ་གྱི་བག་སྒྲིབ་ཐམས་ཅད་སྲེག་གཏོར་དག་པར་བསམ་ལ། གནམ་ལ་མཆོངས་པ་དང་ཕྱི་རྗེང་གཉིས་ཀྱིས་འཕོངས་ལ་བརྡེག་གེན་མདུན་དུ་[343]བདུན་རྒྱབ་ཏུ་ཕྱི་ལ་འཁོར་ནས་ལན་བདུན་མཆོངས་རྒྱུག་བྱའོ།

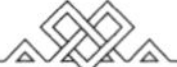

35. Disciplining and Loosening the Channels

Standing, hold your waist with both hands, thumbs pointing forward. Visualize the three channels, six wheels, and the drops of method and wisdom as follows: at the crown an *A*, at the throat an *Om*, at the heart a *Hung*, at the wheel of the soles of the feet a *Yam*, at the secret wheel a *Ram*, and at the navel a *Kham*. Then, the fire of the *tummo* heats the channel-elements. The three syllables *A*, *Om*, and *Hung* melt into light and become the three drops, white, red, and blue respectively, and they dissolve in the *Yam* at the soles of the feet. From the *Yam* a wind moves. From the *Ram* a fire blazes. From the *Kham* nectar falls. From that, imagine that wind and fire emerge as a golden light, and all the propensities and obscurations of the three times are incinerated, dispersed, and purified. While jumping upward, strike the buttocks with both heels. Go forward seven times, then turn and jump back seven times.

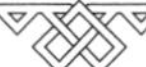

།འཁྲུལ་འཁོར་གསུམ་པོ་འདི་ཡང་སྟོན་ཆེན་པོས་སྲས་འབུམ་རྗེ་འོད་ལ་གསུངས། ཡོན་ཏན་ནི་ནད་རིགས་ཀུན་དང་འབྱུང་བའི་རྐྱེན་ཕྱི་ནང་གེགས་ཐམས་ཅད་ལས་གྲོལ། རྩ་རླུང་ཐིག་ལེའི་སྐྱོན་ཀུན་སེལ། རླུང་ལྷ་གནད་དུ་ཚུད། བང་མགྱོགས་བདེ་དྲོད་འབར་འབྱུང་བཞི་ལ་རང་དབང་ཐོབ། རྟོག་ཚོགས་འགྱུ་བ་རང་སར་སངས། བདེ་གསལ་མི་རྟོག་པའི་ཉམས་འཆར་རོ།

These three magical movements were spoken by Yangton Chenpo to his son Bumje Ö.

Benefits

One is liberated from all outer and inner obstacles: the cooperative conditions of the elements and all kinds of diseases. All defects of the channels, winds, and drops are cleared. The five winds penetrate the vital points. One obtains mastery of speed-walking, the blazing of blissful warmth, and the four elements. The motion of the hordes of thoughts naturally clears and nonconceptual experiences of bliss and clarity arise. An experience of nonconceptual bliss and clarity arises.

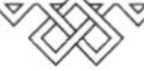

།སོ་དྲུག་པ་རྒྱ་མོ་དར་འཐག་དང་པོ་ནི། འདུག་ལ་རྐང་པ་གཉིས་མདུན་དུ་བཞག་ལག་པ་གཡས་པས་རྐང་གཡས་པོལ་ཚིགས་ལ་བཟུང་། ལག་གཡོན་རྐང་པ་གཡོན་པའི་སྐྱིད་ཁུག་ནང་ནས་ཕྱིར་བརྟོན་ལ་རྐང་པའི་མཐེབ་མོ་ལ་བཟུང་ནས་ནང་དུ་[344]བདུན་ཕྱི་ཏུ་བདུན་བསྐོར། དེ་བཞིན་གཡས་གཡོན་བརྗེ་བར་ཤེས་པར་བྱ།

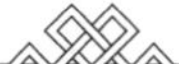

36. Chinese Woman Weaving Silk, Part One

Sitting down, place both legs in front. With the right hand hold the right ankle. Drawing the left hand out from the inside of the kneepit of the left leg, hold the second toe. Then, rotate the leg seven times inward and seven times outward. Like this, understand that the right and the left should be switched.

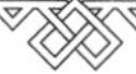

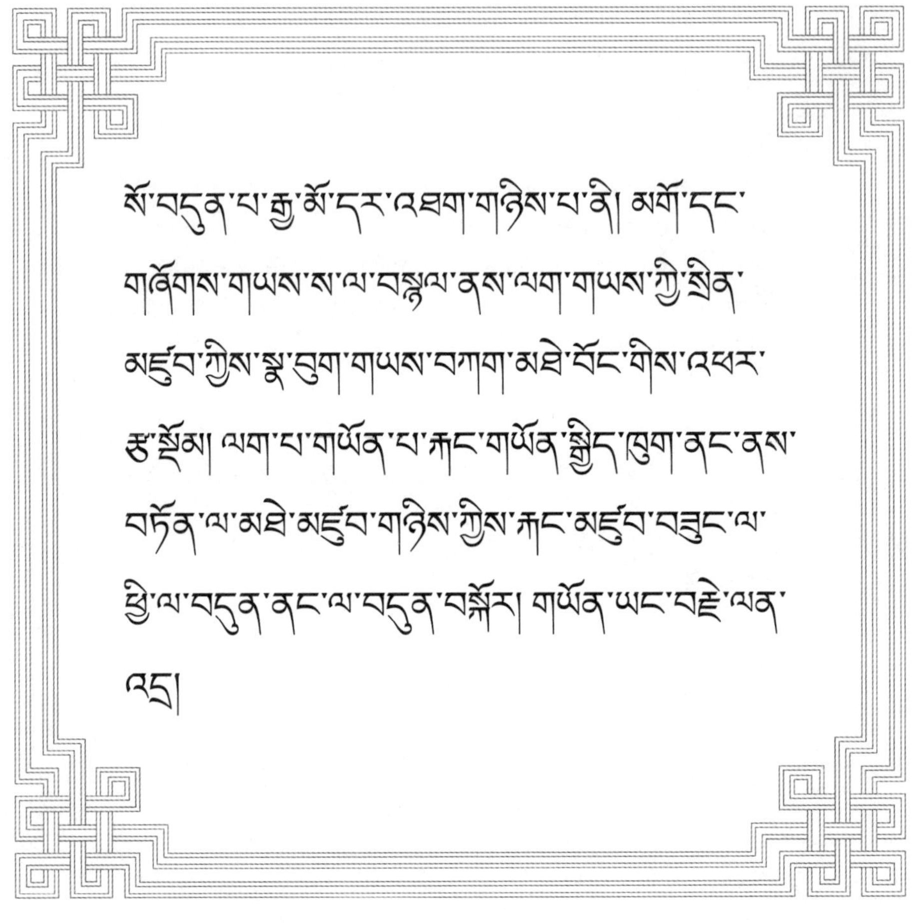

སོ་བདུན་པ་རྒྱ་མོ་དར་འཐག་གཉིས་པ་ནི། མགོ་དང་གཞོགས་གཡས་ས་ལ་བསྙལ་ནས་ལག་གཡས་ཀྱི་སྲིན་མཛུབ་ཀྱིས་སྣ་བུག་གཡས་བཀག་མཐེ་བོང་གིས་འཕར་རྩ་སྡོམ། ལག་པ་གཡོན་པ་རྐང་གཡོན་སྒྲིད་ཁུག་ནང་ནས་བཏོན་ལ་མཐེ་མཛུབ་གཉིས་ཀྱིས་རྐང་མཛུབ་བཟུང་ལ་ཕྱི་ལ་བདུན་ནང་ལ་བདུན་བསྐོར། གཡོན་ཡང་བརྗེ་ལན་འདྲ།

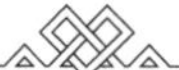

37. Chinese Woman Weaving Silk, Part Two

Lie with your head and right side of body on the ground. Then, with the ring finger of your right hand close the right nostril. With your thumb press the carotid artery. Drawing the left arm inside the left kneepit, with both the thumb and forefinger hold the second toe. Rotate the leg seven times outward and seven times inward. Repeat, switching the right with the left.

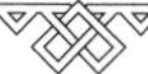

སོ་བརྒྱད་པ་རྒྱ་མོ་དར་འཕག་གསུམ་པ་ནི། ཙོག་པུར་
འདུག་ལ་ལག་གཉིས་རྐང་པའི་བར་ནས་བརྐྱང་ལ་རྐང་
མཐེ་གཉིས་ལ་བཟུང་། ཕྱི་འཕོངས་ས་ལ་བཙུག་ནས་རྐང་
ལག་ཙུང་ཟད་བཀུག་ལ་ཕྱི་རྗིང་གཉིས་རེས་མོས་དཔྱི་
ཏབ་ལ་ལན་བདུན་རེ་རྒྱོབ་པའོ། །གཟུགས་བཞི་གསིགས་
སྦྲུགས་སོགས་འདྲའོ།

38. Chinese Woman Weaving Silk, Part Three

Sitting on the floor, extend both arms between the legs and hold the big toes of both feet. Planting the outside of the buttocks on the ground, with the legs and arms slightly lifted, project the two ankles toward the hips, repeating seven times with each heel. Shudder and shake the four limbs, and so forth, same as before.

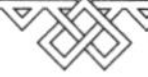

[345]ཡོན་ཏན་ནི། དང་པོ་གཡོན་གྱི་རྩ་སྒོ་འབྱེད་ཅིང་ཤེས་རབ་འཕེལ། མོ་རླུང་གནད་དུ་ཚུད་ཅིང་འགྲོ་རྒོད་ཞི། གཉིས་པས་གཡས་ཀྱི་རྩ་སྒོ་འགག་ཅིང་ཉོན་མོངས་རྒྱུན་ལམ་ཆད། རྩུབ་རླུང་རང་དབང་ཐོབ་ཅིང་བྱིང་རྨུགས་སངས། གསུམ་པས་དབུ་མའི་རྩ་སྒོ་འབྱེད་ཅིང་མ་ནིང་རླུང་ལ་འབྱོངས། སྣང་སེམས་རང་དབང་ཐོབ་ཅིང་མི་རྟོག་ཡེ་ཤེས་འཆར། ཞེས་སོ།

Benefits

[From *Quintessential Oral Instructions*:]

> The first part of the "Chinese woman weaving silk" magical movement opens the door of the left channel, and wisdom increases. The female wind penetrates the vital points and pacifies agitation and the proliferation of thoughts.
>
> The second closes the door of the right channel and cuts off the continuous flow of mental afflictions. Mastery over the coarse winds is obtained and torpor and dullness are dispelled.
>
> The third opens the door of the central channel and trains the neutral wind. Mastery of appearances and mind is obtained, and nonconceptual primordial wisdom arises.

སོར་དགུ་པ་ནོར་བུ་འཕར་ལེན་ནི། སེམས་དཔའི་སྐྱིལ་ཀྲུང་བཅའ་ལ་ལག་པའི་སོར་མོ་བསྣོལ་ནས་མཐེབ་མོ་གཉིས་གཤིབས་ཏེ་རྩེ་མོ་སྦྲད། མཐེ་བོང་གཡོན་གྱིས་གཡས་མནན་ལ་བསྣོལ་ཏེ་ལག་གཉིས་ཤད་ཀྱིས་བརྐྱང་ཞིང་ནང་དུ་བཀུག་མཐེ་བོང་རྒྱབ་ཚོགས་བྲང་གི་གཡས་གཡོན་དཀྱིལ་དང་། ཁྱད་པར་གང་ན་བའི་སྟེང་དུ་རྒྱོབ་པ་དང་ཕཊཿ[346]སྒྲ་འདོན་པ་དུས་མཉམ་དུ་ཐེ་མང་བྱ་བ་དང་། གསེགས་སྐྱུགས་ཧ་ཕཊཿསོགས་ནི་འཁྲུལ་འཁོར་ཀུན་ལ་འགྲེས།

39. Bouncing Jewel

Assume the bodhisattva posture, interlacing the fingers of the hands, with the two forefingers parallel, fingertips touching, interleave the thumbs, the left thumb pressing the right. Extend both hands straight and then bend them inward, hitting with the back joints of the thumbs, the right, left, and center of the chest. Strike any place and simultaneously vocalize the *phat* sound as many times as possible. Then, stir and shake with *ha phat* and so forth; those should be integrated with all of the magical movements.

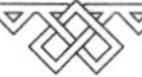

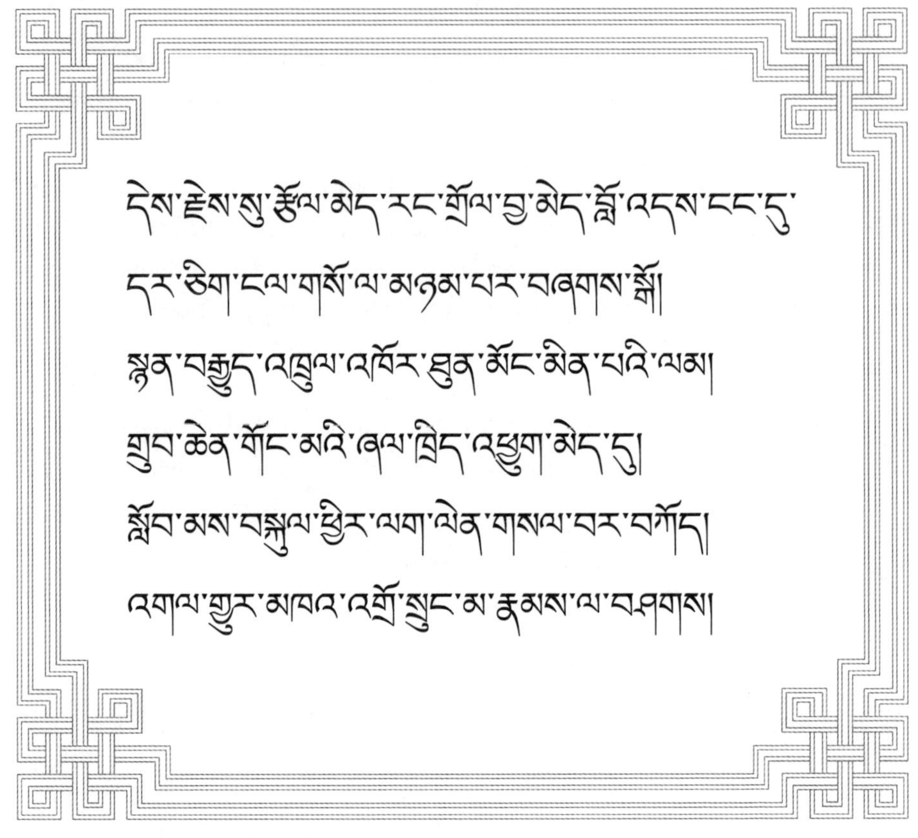

དེས་རྗེས་སུ་རྩོལ་མེད་རང་གྲོལ་བྱ་མེད་བློ་འདས་ངང་དུ་
དར་ཅིག་ངལ་གསོ་ལ་མཉམ་པར་བཞགས་སྐོ།
སྙན་བརྒྱུད་འཁྲུལ་འཁོར་ཐུན་མོང་མིན་པའི་ལམ།
གྲུབ་ཆེན་གོང་མའི་ཞལ་ཁྲིད་འཕྲུག་མེད་དུ།
སློབ་མས་བསྐུལ་ཕྱིར་ལག་ལེན་གསལ་བར་བཀོད།
འགལ་འགྱུར་མཁའ་འགྲོ་སྲུང་མ་རྣམས་ལ་བཤགས།

Concluding Advice

Thus, in conclusion, rest easefully for a moment in a meditatitive equipoise, a state that is effortless, naturally liberated, free of action, and beyond the intellect.

Colophon

Due to the request of my student, I composed with clarity this guidebook,
an unmistaken oral guide of the teachings of the earlier Great Accomplished Ones,
to the uncommon path of magical movements of the aural tradition of Zhang Zhung.
I confess my errors to the *dakinis* and guardians.

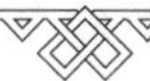

ཞེས་པ་འདིའང་དབྲ་ཡི་དཔོན་པོ་རྣམ་རྒྱལ་གྲགས་
པ་དང་དབྲ་སློབ་ཚུལ་ཁྲིམས་རྒྱལ་མཚན་གཉིས་ཀྱིས།
གདམས་པ་ཟབ་མོ་འདི་འདྲ་ཞལ་ཁྲིད་འཇོལ་དོགས་དང་
བརྒྱུད་པ་ཆད་ན་ཕོངས་སེམས་ཆེ་བར་སྣམ་ནས། ཞལ་
ཁྲིད་བཞིན་ཡིག་ལམ་ལ་བཀོད་དགོས་ཀྱིས་བསྐུལ་མ་
བྱུང་བ་བཞིན་ཤར་རྫའི་བྱ་བྲལ་བཀྲ་ཤིས་རྒྱལ་མཚན་
གྱིས་གསུང་དྲུང་ལྷུན་པོ་བདེ་ཆེན་རི་ཁྲོད་དུ་བཀོད་པ་
འདིས་ཀྱང་རླུང་སེམས་ཟུང་འཇུག་གི་རྣལ་འབྱོར་པས་རི་
སུལ་གང་ན་ཉམས་རྟོགས་ཁྱད་པར་ཅན་ལ་འཁྲུངས་པའི་
རྐྱེན་དུ་གྱུར་ཅིག །སརྦ་མངྒལཾ།

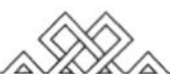

Furthermore, a chief of the *dra* clan, Namgyal Dragpa, and a student of the *dra* clan, Tsultrim Gyaltsen, had the strong reflection that for a profound instruction like this, if the oral guidance became confused and the lineage was broken, it would be a great loss. Due to the need to put into writing the oral guidance, the exhortation to compose arose. Accordingly, Shardza Jadral Tashi Gyaltsen composed this in the Yungdrung Dechen Lhunpo mountain hermitage. Through this, and through the yogi's fusion of wind and mind, amidst these mountains, may they become the conditions for giving birth to extraordinary experiences and realizations.

Sarva mangalam

This translation from Tibetan into English was completed by Kurt Keutzer and Alejandro Chaoul.

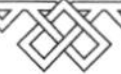

APPENDIX 2

Shardza's *Channels-and-Winds Prayer*

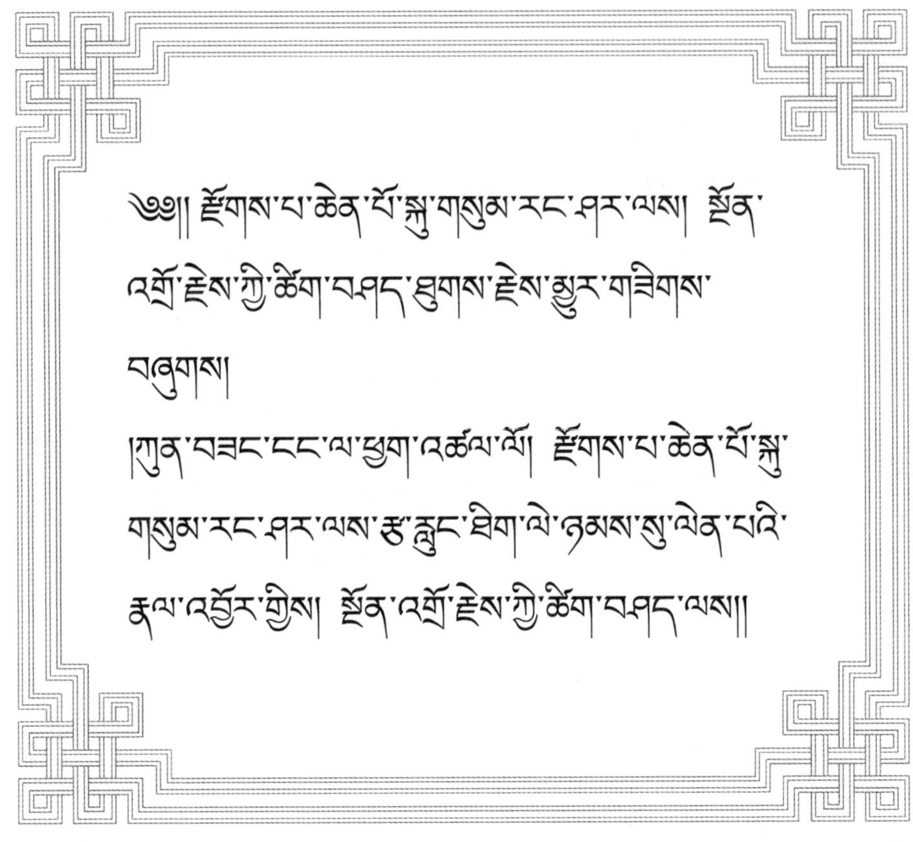

༄༅། །རྫོགས་པ་ཆེན་པོ་སྐུ་གསུམ་རང་ཤར་ལས། སྔོན་འགྲོ་རྗེས་ཀྱི་ཚིག་བཤད་ཐུགས་རྗེས་སྐུར་གཟིགས་བཞུགས།

།ཀུན་བཟང་དང་ལ་ཕྱག་འཚལ་ལོ། རྫོགས་པ་ཆེན་པོ་སྐུ་གསུམ་རང་ཤར་ལས་རྩ་རླུང་ཐིག་ལེ་ཉམས་སུ་ལེན་པའི་རྣལ་འབྱོར་གྱིས། སྔོན་འགྲོ་རྗེས་ཀྱི་ཚིག་བཤད་ལས།།

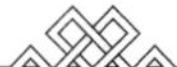

I prostrate to the state of Kuntuzangpo. From the text *Dzogchen: The Natural Arising of the Three Enlightened Bodies* by Shardza Tashi Gyaltsen: preliminary and concluding chants for the yogi who engages in the practices of *tsa*, *lung*, and *thiklé*.

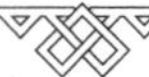

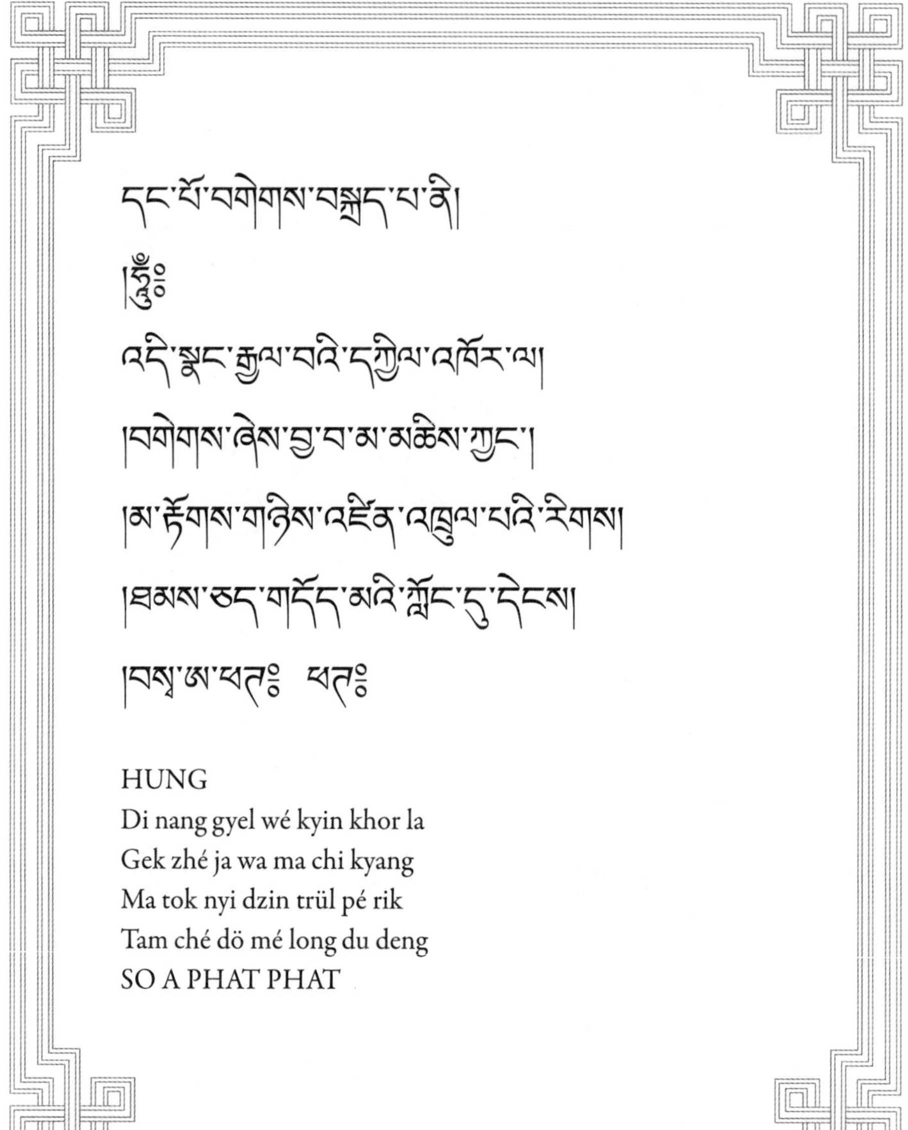

དང་པོ་བགེགས་བསྐྲད་པ་ནི།

།ཧཱུྃ༔

འདི་སྣང་རྒྱལ་བའི་དཀྱིལ་འཁོར་ལ།

།བགེགས་ཞེས་བྱ་བ་མ་མཆིས་ཀྱང་།

།མ་རྟོགས་གཉིས་འཛིན་འཁྲུལ་པའི་རིགས།

།ཐམས་ཅད་གདོད་མའི་ཀློང་དུ་དེངས།

།སྭ་ཨ་ཕཊ༔ ཕཊ༔

HUNG
Di nang gyel wé kyin khor la
Gek zhé ja wa ma chi kyang
Ma tok nyi dzin trül pé rik
Tam ché dö mé long du deng
SO A PHAT PHAT

First, expelling obstacles:

HUNG
Even the word "obstacle" does not exist,
Here, in the mandala of the Victor's appearances.
All these aspects of lack of realization, grasping at delusion,
Vanish into the primordial expanse.
SO A PHAT PHAT

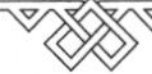

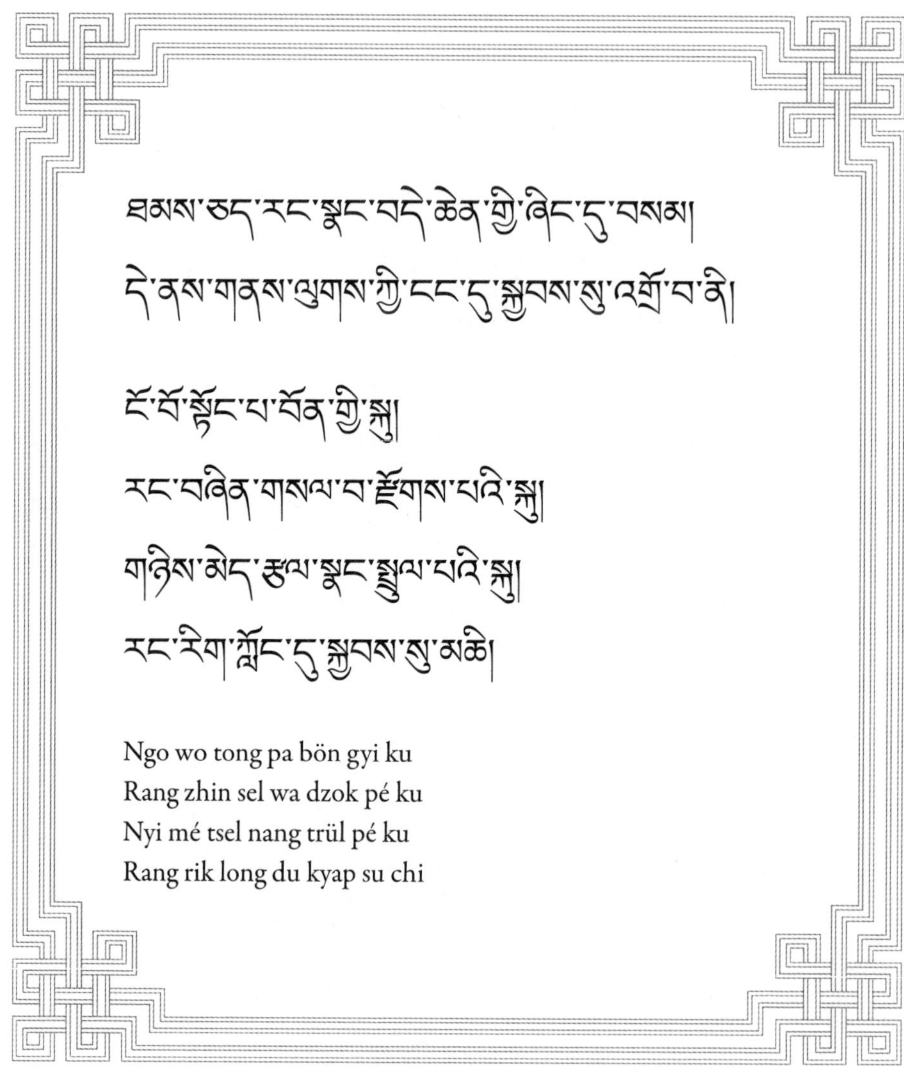

ཐམས་ཅད་རང་སྣང་བདེ་ཆེན་གྱི་ཞིང་དུ་བསམ།
དེ་ནས་གནས་ལུགས་ཀྱི་ངང་དུ་སྐྱབས་སུ་འགྲོ་བ་ནི།

ངོ་བོ་སྟོང་པ་བོན་གྱི་སྐུ།
རང་བཞིན་གསལ་བ་རྫོགས་པའི་སྐུ།
གཉིས་མེད་རྩལ་སྣང་སྤྲུལ་པའི་སྐུ།
རང་རིག་ཀློང་དུ་སྐྱབས་སུ་མཆི།

Ngo wo tong pa bön gyi ku
Rang zhin sel wa dzok pé ku
Nyi mé tsel nang trül pé ku
Rang rik long du kyap su chi

(Think that everything is a realm of intensely blissful natural appearances. Then, go for refuge in the continuity of the natural state.)

Refuge

In the empty essence, the *bön ku*,
In the luminous nature, the *dzok ku*,
In the nonduality of dynamic energy and appearances, the *tulku*,
In the expanse of innate self-awareness,
I take refuge.

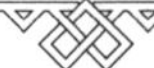

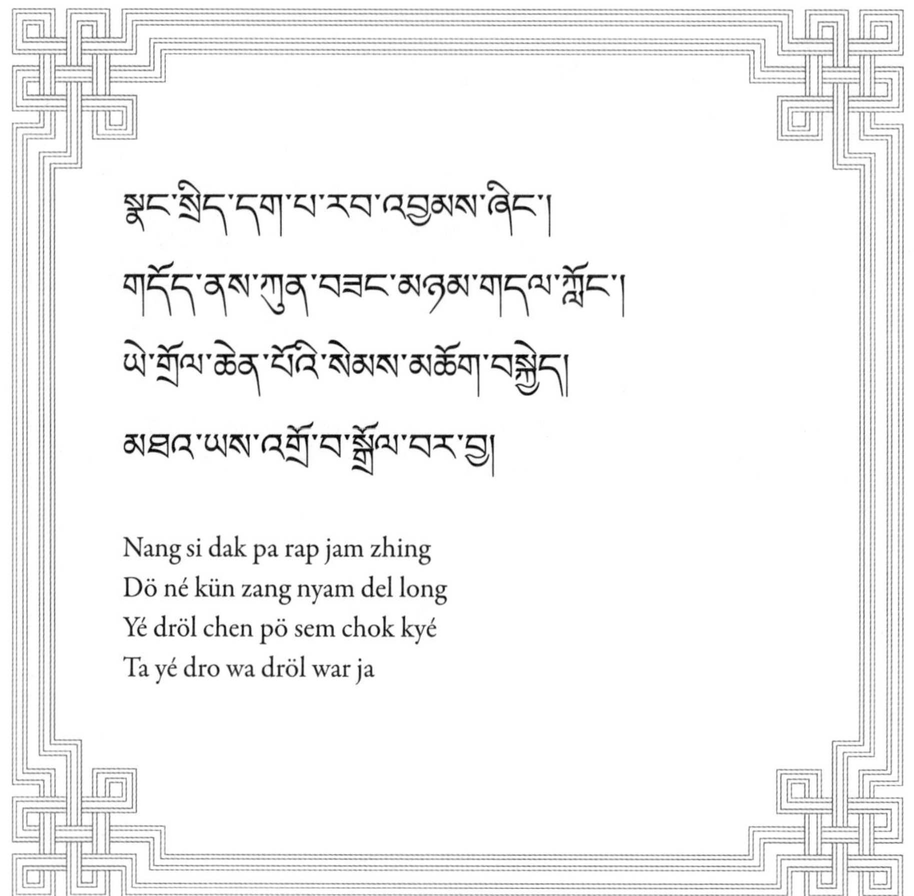

སྣང་སྲིད་དག་པ་རབ་འབྱམས་ཞིང་།
གདོད་ནས་ཀུན་བཟང་མཉམ་གདལ་ཀློང་།
ཡེ་གྲོལ་ཆེན་པོའི་སེམས་མཆོག་བསྐྱེད།
མཐའ་ཡས་འགྲོ་བ་སྒྲོལ་བར་བྱ།

Nang si dak pa rap jam zhing
Dö né kün zang nyam del long
Yé dröl chen pö sem chok kyé
Ta yé dro wa dröl war ja

Bodhicitta

This immeasurable realm of pure apparent existence,
Is primordially equal with Kuntuzangpo, the pervasive expanse.
I generate the supreme mind of the great primordial liberation.
May I liberate infinite sentient beings.

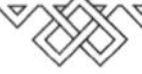

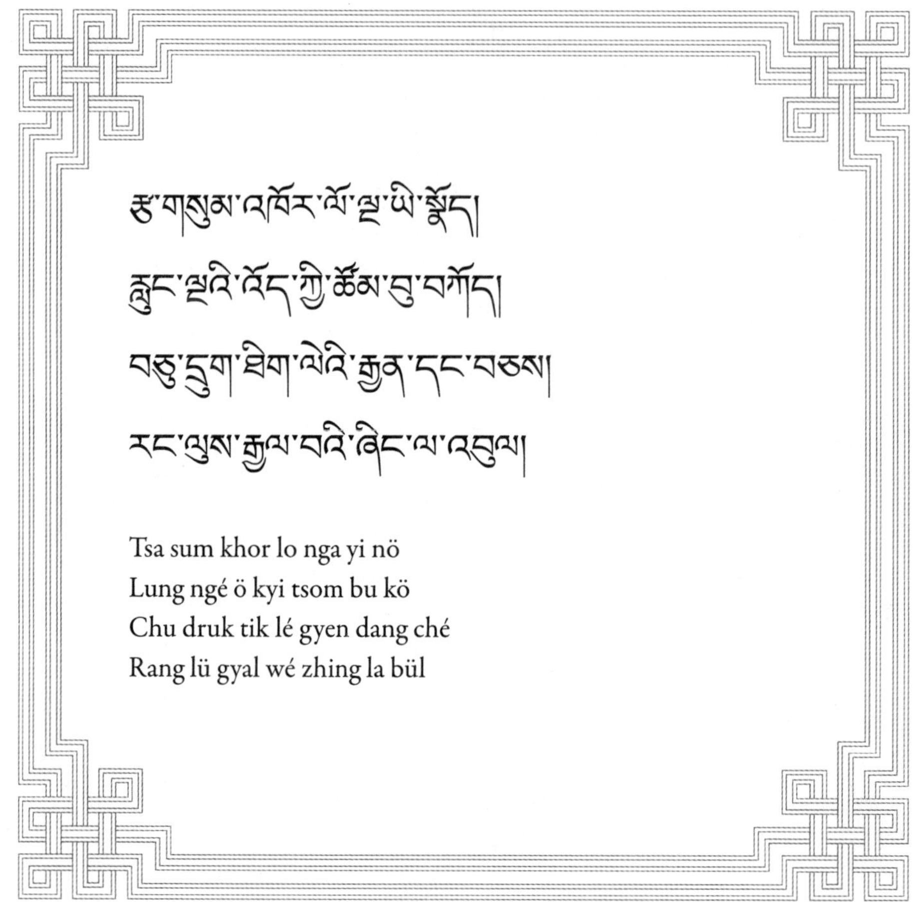

རྩ་གསུམ་འཁོར་ལོ་ལྔ་ཡི་སྣོད།
རླུང་ལྔའི་འོད་ཀྱི་ཚོམ་བུ་བཀོད།
བཅུ་དྲུག་ཐིག་ལེའི་རྒྱན་དང་བཅས།
རང་ལུས་རྒྱལ་བའི་ཞིང་ལ་འབུལ།

Tsa sum khor lo nga yi nö
Lung ngé ö kyi tsom bu kö
Chu druk tik lé gyen dang ché
Rang lü gyal wé zhing la bül

Offering the mandala of the actual *tsa* and *lung*.

The vessel of three *tsa* and five *khorlo*,
Arrayed with the heaps of light of the five *lung*,
Together with the ornaments of the sixteen *thiklé*,
I offer this mandala of my body to the realm of the Victorious Ones.

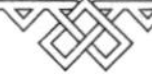

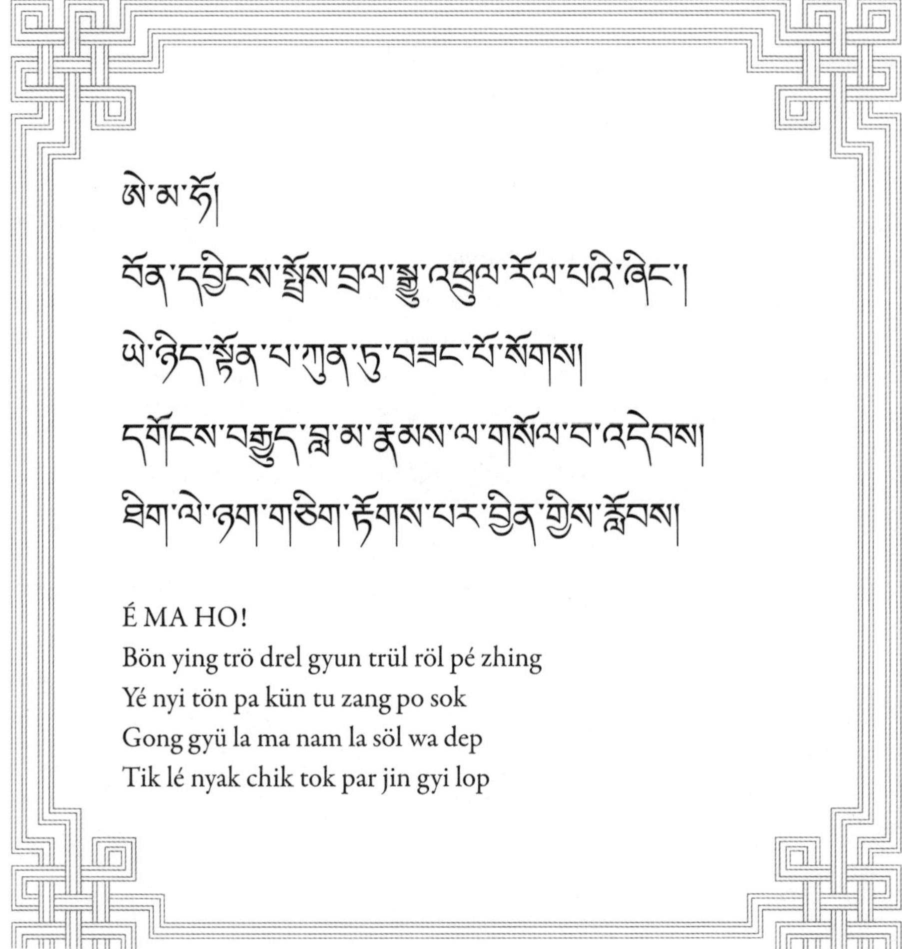

ཨེ་མ་ཧོ།

བོན་དབྱིངས་སྤྲོས་བྲལ་སྒྱུ་འཕྲུལ་རོལ་པའི་ཞིང་།

ཡེ་ཉིད་སྟོན་པ་ཀུན་ཏུ་བཟང་པོ་སོགས།

དགོངས་བརྒྱུད་བླ་མ་རྣམས་ལ་གསོལ་བ་འདེབས།

ཐིག་ལེ་ཉག་གཅིག་རྟོགས་པར་བྱིན་གྱིས་རློབས།

É MA HO!
Bön ying trö drel gyun trül röl pé zhing
Yé nyi tön pa kün tu zang po sok
Gong gyü la ma nam la söl wa dep
Tik lé nyak chik tok par jin gyi lop

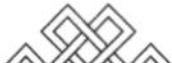

(Then, pray to the masters of the mental, symbolic, and aural-transmission lineages:)

É MA HO!
In the unelaborated space of *bön*, the realm of the play of magical
emanations,
Is the primordial teacher, Kuntuzangpo and others,
I pray to the masters of the direct mind-transmission lineage:
Bless me to realize the single sphere.

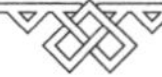

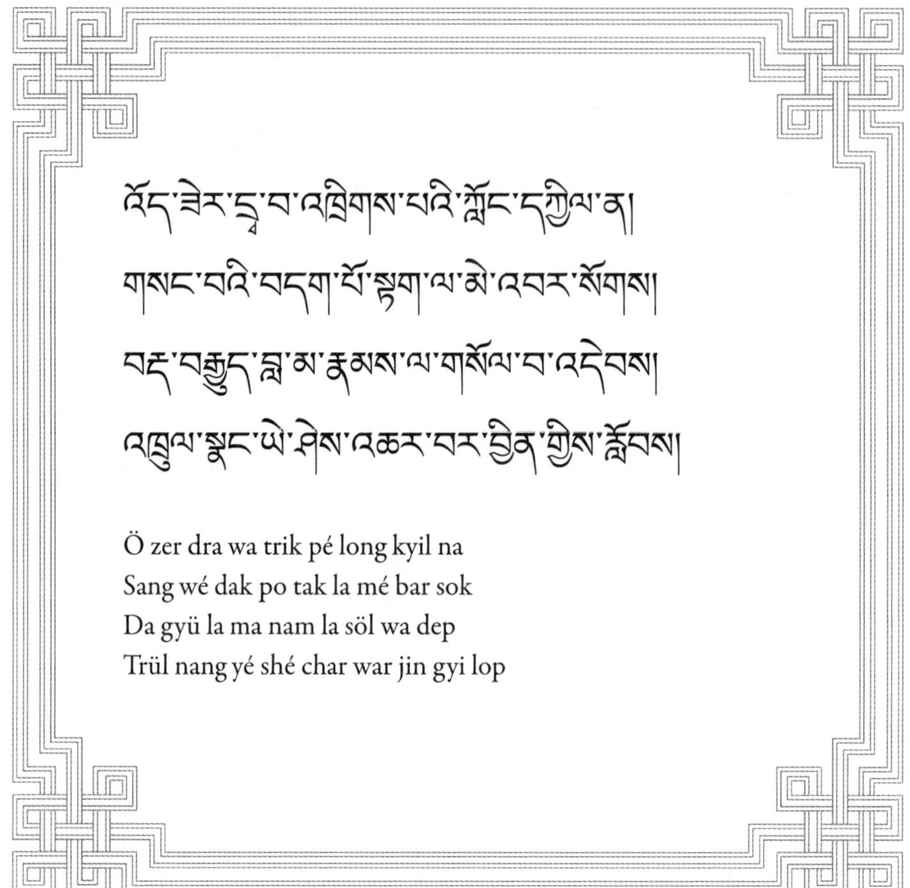

འོད་ཟེར་དྲྭ་བ་འཁྲིགས་པའི་ཀློང་དཀྱིལ་ན།
གསང་བའི་བདག་པོ་སྟག་ལ་མེ་འབར་སོགས།
བརྡ་བརྒྱུད་བླ་མ་རྣམས་ལ་གསོལ་བ་འདེབས།
འཁྲུལ་སྣང་ཡེ་ཤེས་འཆར་བར་བྱིན་གྱིས་རློབས།

Ö zer dra wa trik pé long kyil na
Sang wé dak po tak la mé bar sok
Da gyü la ma nam la söl wa dep
Trül nang yé shé char war jin gyi lop

In the center of an expanse of a flashing web of light rays,
Is the lord of secrets, Takla Mébar, and others.
I pray to the masters of the lineage of symbols:
Bless me that deluded appearances will arise as primordial wisdom.

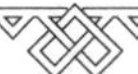

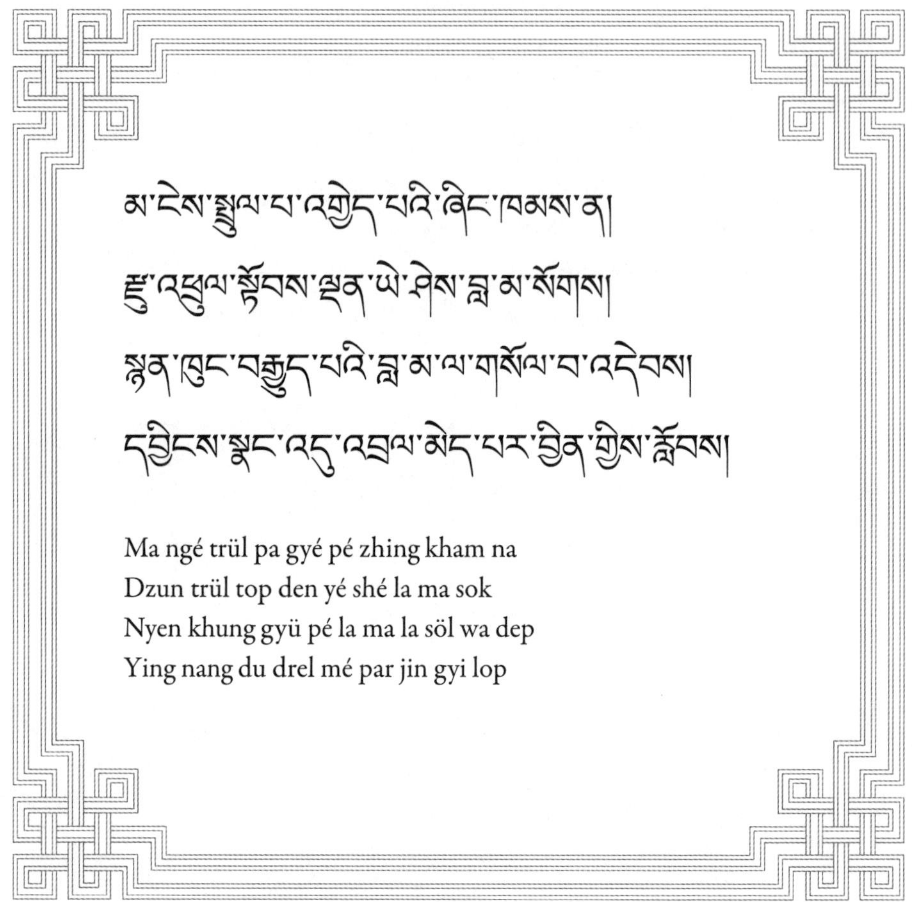

མ་ངེས་སྤྲུལ་པ་འགྱེད་པའི་ཞིང་ཁམས་ན།
རྫུ་འཕྲུལ་སྟོབས་ལྡན་ཡེ་ཤེས་བླ་མ་སོགས།
སྙན་ཁུང་བརྒྱུད་པའི་བླ་མ་ལ་གསོལ་བ་འདེབས།
དབྱིངས་སྣང་འདུ་འབྲལ་མེད་པར་བྱིན་གྱིས་རློབས།

Ma ngé trül pa gyé pé zhing kham na
Dzun trül top den yé shé la ma sok
Nyen khung gyü pé la ma la söl wa dep
Ying nang du drel mé par jin gyi lop

Within a pure realm that issues forth innumerable emanations,
Is the powerful master Dzutrul Yeshé, and others,
I pray to the lamas of the aural lineage:
Bless me to recognize appearances and space as inseparable.

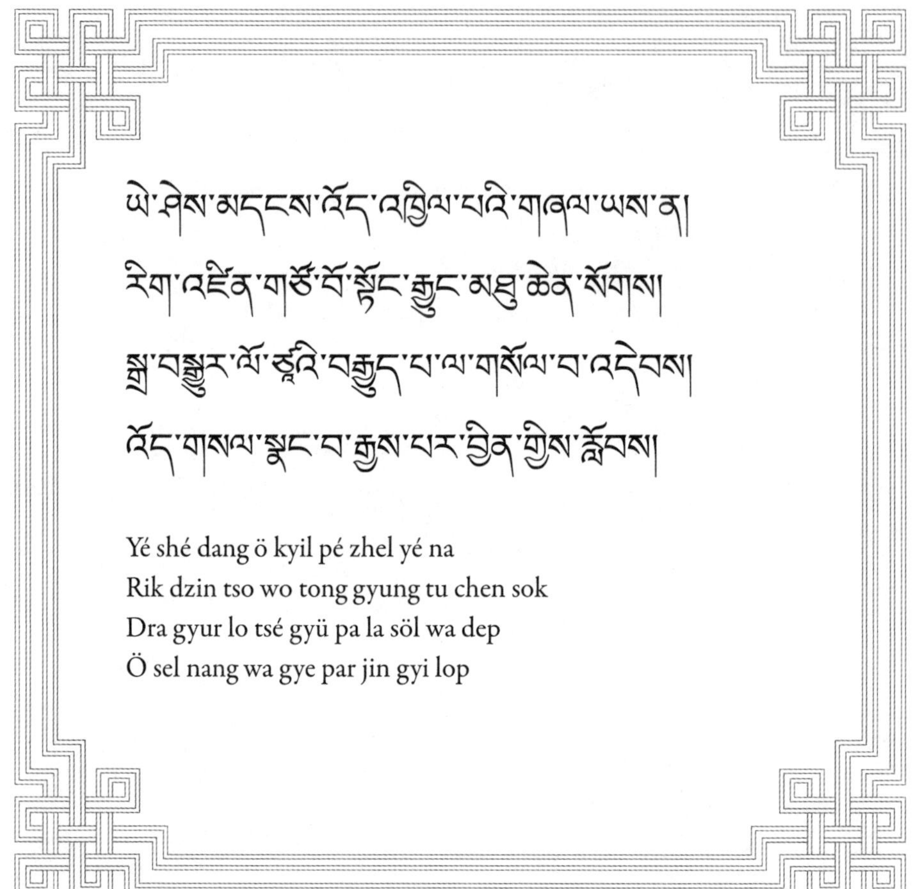

ཡེ་ཤེས་མདངས་འོད་འཁྱིལ་པའི་གཞལ་ཡས་ན།
རིག་འཛིན་གཙོ་བོ་སྟོང་རྒྱུང་མཐུ་ཆེན་སོགས།
སྒྲ་བསྒྱུར་ལོ་ཙཱའི་བརྒྱུད་པ་ལ་གསོལ་བ་འདེབས།
འོད་གསལ་སྣང་བ་རྒྱས་པར་བྱིན་གྱིས་རློབས།

Yé shé dang ö kyil pé zhel yé na
Rik dzin tso wo tong gyung tu chen sok
Dra gyur lo tsé gyü pa la söl wa dep
Ö sel nang wa gye par jin gyi lop

Within a celestial palace of spirals of radiant wisdom,
Is the principal knowledge holder, Tong Gyung Tuchen, and others.
I pray to the lineage of translators:
Bless me that appearances of clear light may increase.

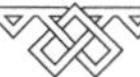

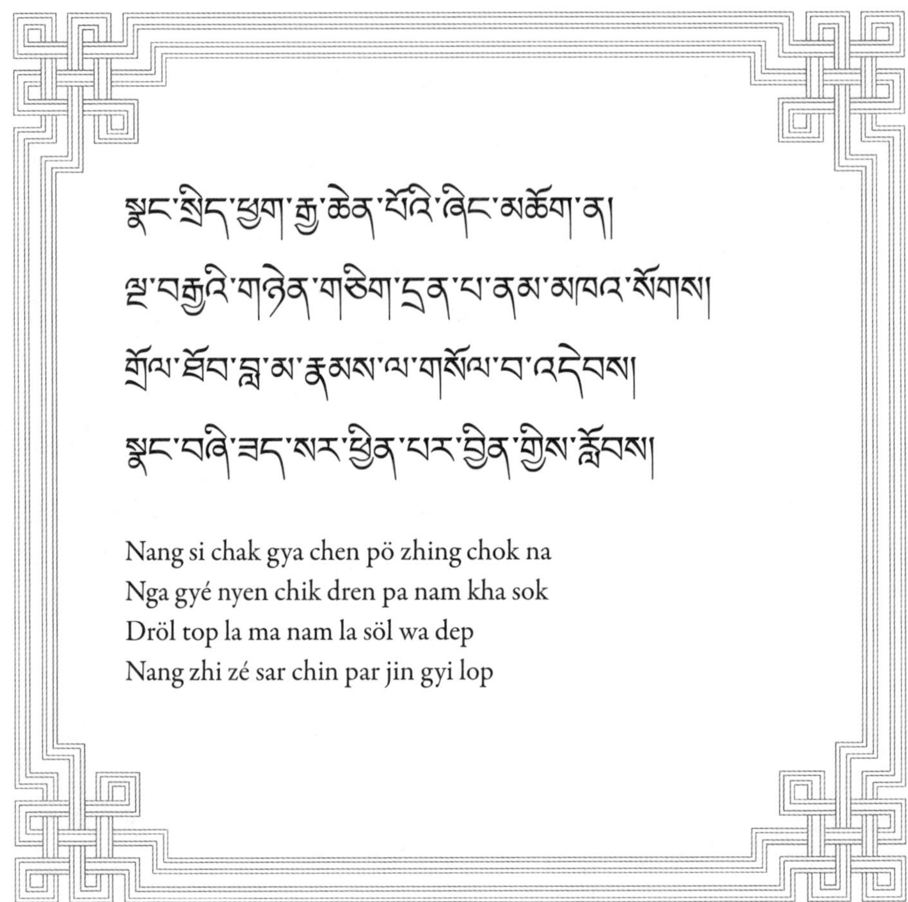

སྣང་སྲིད་ཕྱག་རྒྱ་ཆེན་པོའི་ཞིང་མཆོག་ན།
ལྔ་བརྒྱའི་གཉེན་གཅིག་དྲན་པ་ནམ་མཁའ་སོགས།
གྲོལ་ཐོབ་བླ་མ་རྣམས་ལ་གསོལ་བ་འདེབས།
སྣང་བཞི་ཟད་སར་ཕྱིན་པར་བྱིན་གྱིས་རློབས།

Nang si chak gya chen pö zhing chok na
Nga gyé nyen chik dren pa nam kha sok
Dröl top la ma nam la söl wa dep
Nang zhi zé sar chin par jin gyi lop

Within apparent existence, the supreme realm of Mahamudra,
Is the single antidote of five hundred previous lives, Drenpa Namkha, and others.
I pray to the lamas who have attained liberation:
Bless me to arrive at the state of the exhaustion of the four appearances.

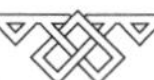

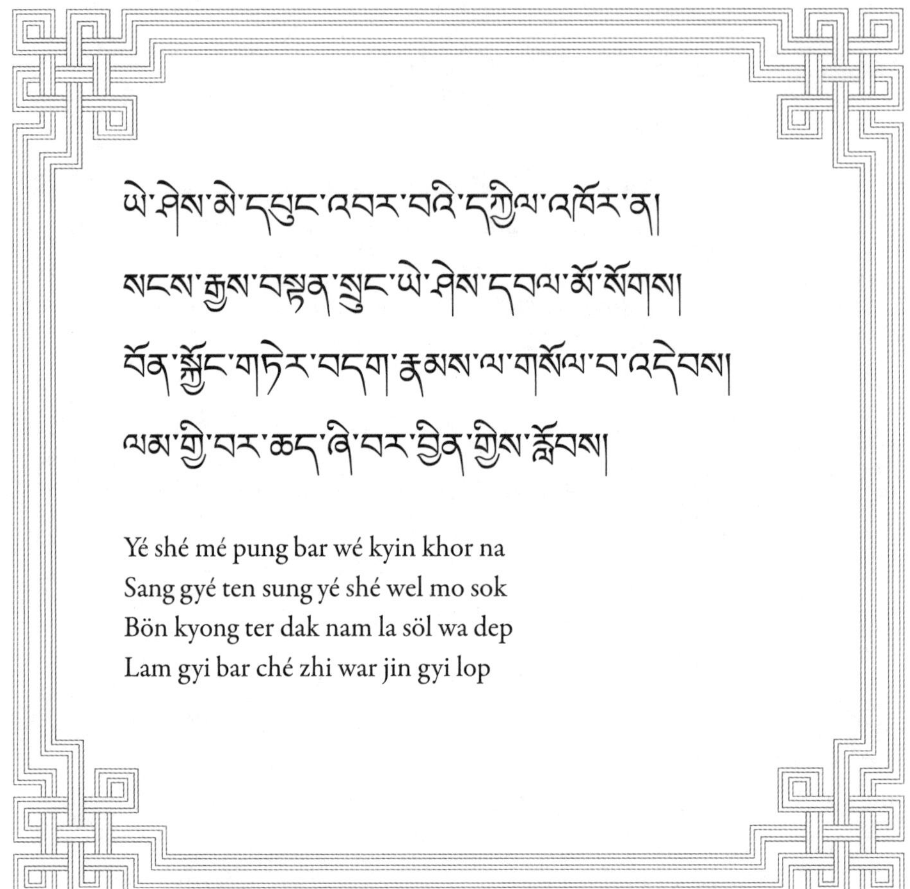

ཡེ་ཤེས་མེ་དཔུང་འབར་བའི་དཀྱིལ་འཁོར་ན།
སངས་རྒྱས་བསྟན་སྲུང་ཡེ་ཤེས་དབལ་མོ་སོགས།
བོན་སྐྱོང་གཏེར་བདག་རྣམས་ལ་གསོལ་བ་འདེབས།
ལམ་གྱི་བར་ཆད་ཞི་བར་བྱིན་གྱིས་རློབས།

Yé shé mé pung bar wé kyin khor na
Sang gyé ten sung yé shé wel mo sok
Bön kyong ter dak nam la söl wa dep
Lam gyi bar ché zhi war jin gyi lop

Within a mandala of a fireball of primordial wisdom
Is the enlightened guardian of the teachings, Yeshé Walmo, and others.
I pray to the guardians of Bön and the lords of *terma*:
Bless me that obstacles to the path are pacified.

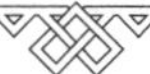

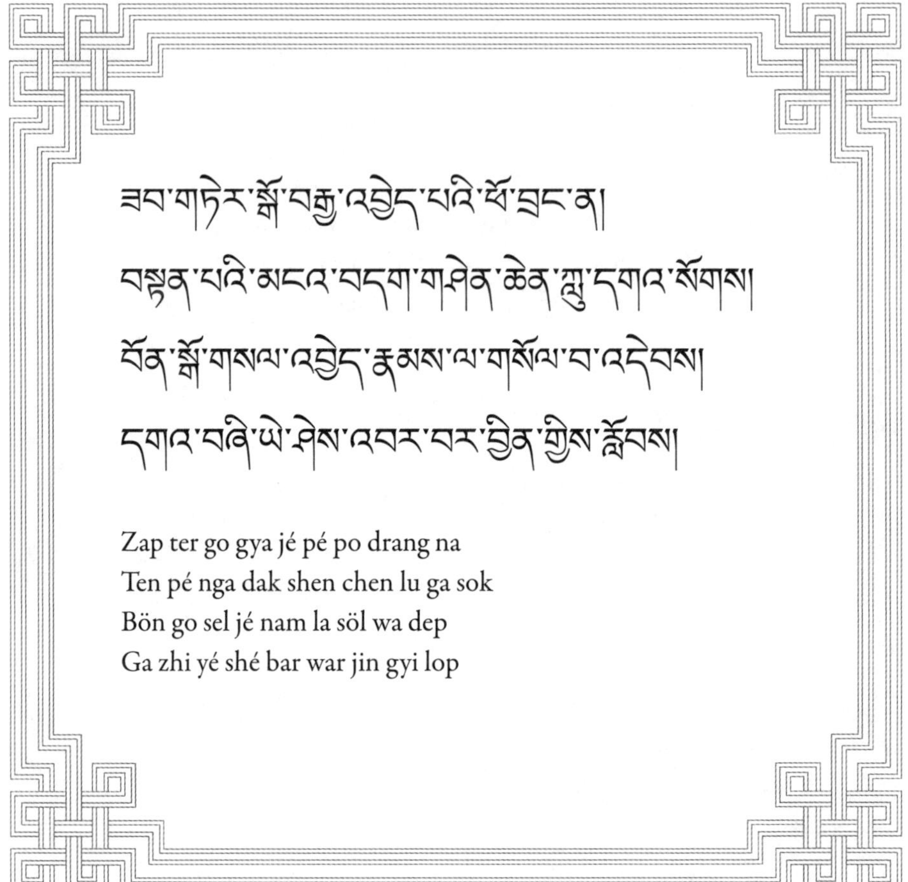

ཟབ་གཏེར་སྒོ་བརྒྱ་འབྱེད་པའི་ཕོ་བྲང་ན།
བསྟན་པའི་མངའ་བདག་གཤེན་ཆེན་ཀླུ་དགའ་སོགས།
བོན་སྒོ་གསལ་འབྱེད་རྣམས་ལ་གསོལ་བ་འདེབས།
དགའ་བཞི་ཡེ་ཤེས་འབར་བར་བྱིན་གྱིས་རློབས།

Zap ter go gya jé pé po drang na
Ten pé nga dak shen chen lu ga sok
Bön go sel jé nam la söl wa dep
Ga zhi yé shé bar war jin gyi lop

In a palace that has many open doors of profound *terma*,
Is the sovereign lord of the teachings, Shenchen Luga, and others.
I pray to those who have opened the door to Bön:
Bless me that the four joys of primordial wisdom blaze.

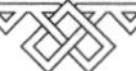

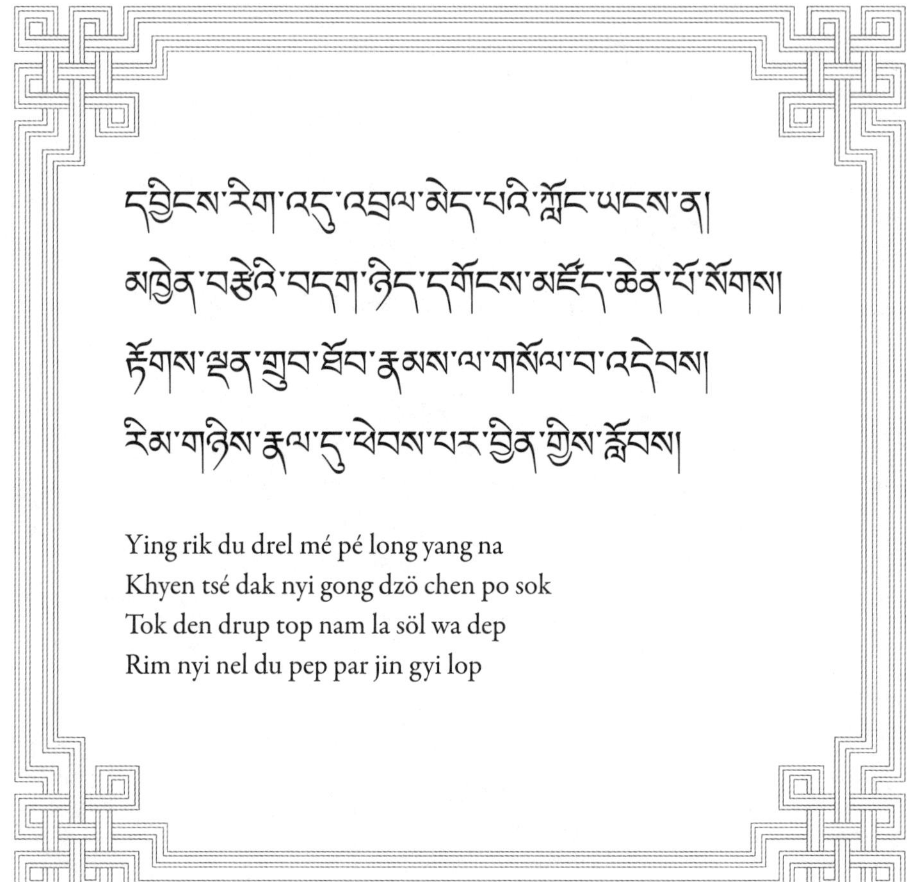

དབྱིངས་རིག་འདུ་འབྲལ་མེད་པའི་ཀློང་ཡངས་ན།
མཁྱེན་བརྩེའི་བདག་ཉིད་དགོངས་མཛོད་ཆེན་པོ་སོགས།
རྟོགས་ལྡན་གྲུབ་ཐོབ་རྣམས་ལ་གསོལ་བ་འདེབས།
རིམ་གཉིས་རྣལ་དུ་ཕེབས་པར་བྱིན་གྱིས་རློབས།

Ying rik du drel mé pé long yang na
Khyen tsé dak nyi gong dzö chen po sok
Tok den drup top nam la söl wa dep
Rim nyi nel du pep par jin gyi lop

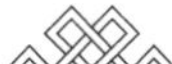

In the vast expanse of the inseparable space and awareness,
Is the personification of knowledge and kindness, Gongdzö Chenpo,
and others.
I pray to the yogis and *siddhas*:
Bless me to be steady in the two stages of development and completion.

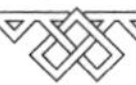

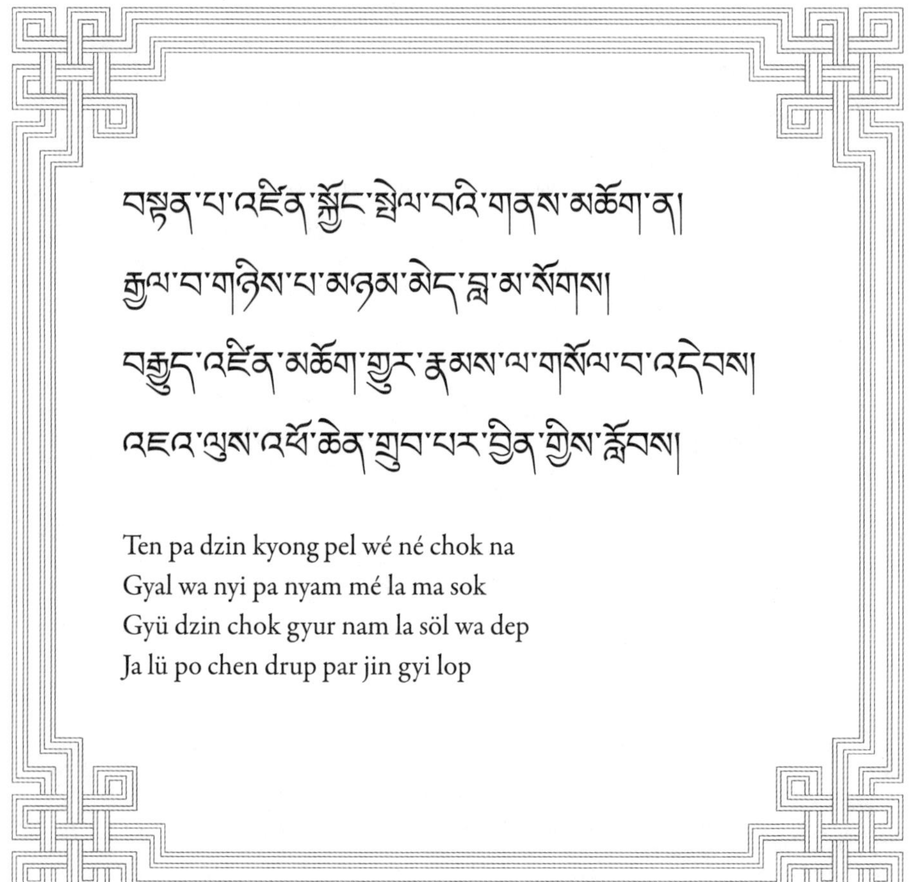

བསྟན་པ་འཛིན་སྐྱོང་སྤེལ་བའི་གནས་མཆོག་ན།
རྒྱལ་བ་གཉིས་པ་མཉམ་མེད་བླ་མ་སོགས།
བརྒྱུད་འཛིན་མཆོག་གྱུར་རྣམས་ལ་གསོལ་བ་འདེབས།
འཇའ་ལུས་འཕོ་ཆེན་གྲུབ་པར་བྱིན་གྱིས་རློབས།

Ten pa dzin kyong pel wé né chok na
Gyal wa nyi pa nyam mé la ma sok
Gyü dzin chok gyur nam la söl wa dep
Ja lü po chen drup par jin gyi lop

In a supreme place, holding, protecting, and spreading the teachings,
Is the second Victor, Nyamé Sherab Gyaltsen, and others.
I pray to the supreme lineage holders:
Bless me to accomplish the great transference of the rainbow body.

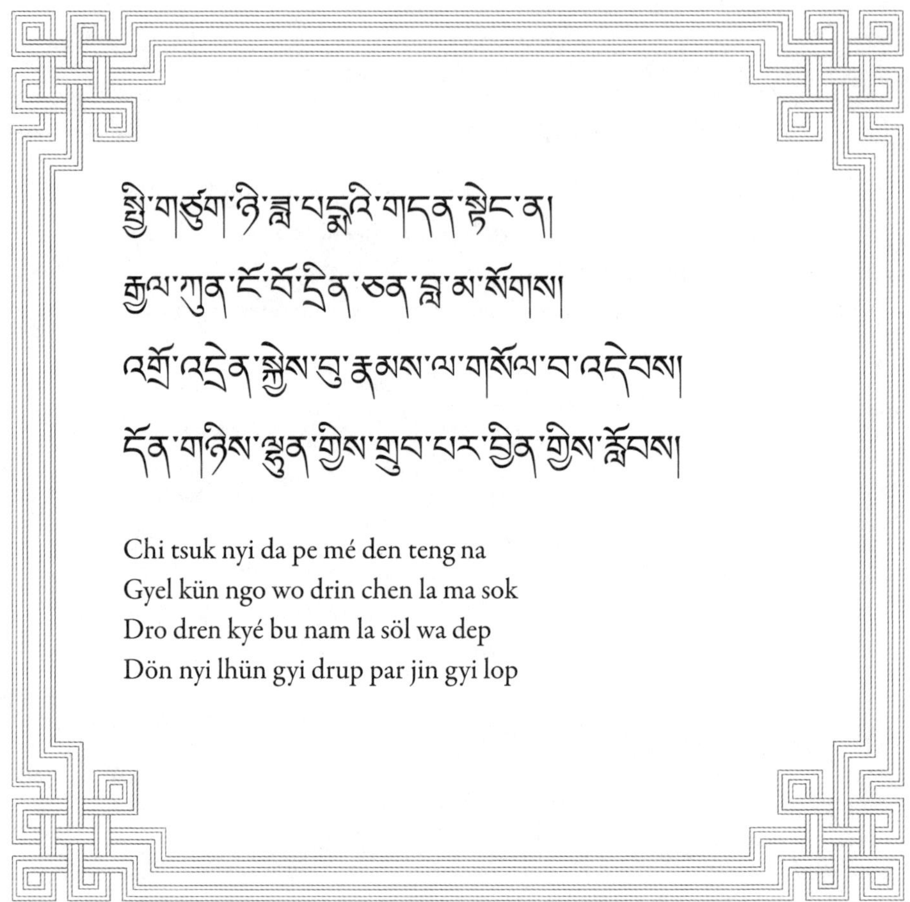

སྤྱི་གཙུག་ཉི་ཟླ་པདྨའི་གདན་སྟེང་ན།
རྒྱལ་ཀུན་ངོ་བོ་དྲིན་ཅན་བླ་མ་སོགས།
འགྲོ་འདྲེན་སྐྱེས་བུ་རྣམས་ལ་གསོལ་བ་འདེབས།
དོན་གཉིས་ལྷུན་གྱིས་གྲུབ་པར་བྱིན་གྱིས་རློབས།

Chi tsuk nyi da pe mé den teng na
Gyel kün ngo wo drin chen la ma sok
Dro dren kyé bu nam la söl wa dep
Dön nyi lhün gyi drup par jin gyi lop

Above the crown of my head, upon a throne of lotus, sun, and moon,
Is the essence of all Victors, my gracious lama, and others.
I pray to those who have the ability to lead beings out of samsara:
Grant your blessings so that I may spontaneously accomplish the two aims of benefitting myself and others.

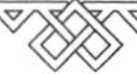

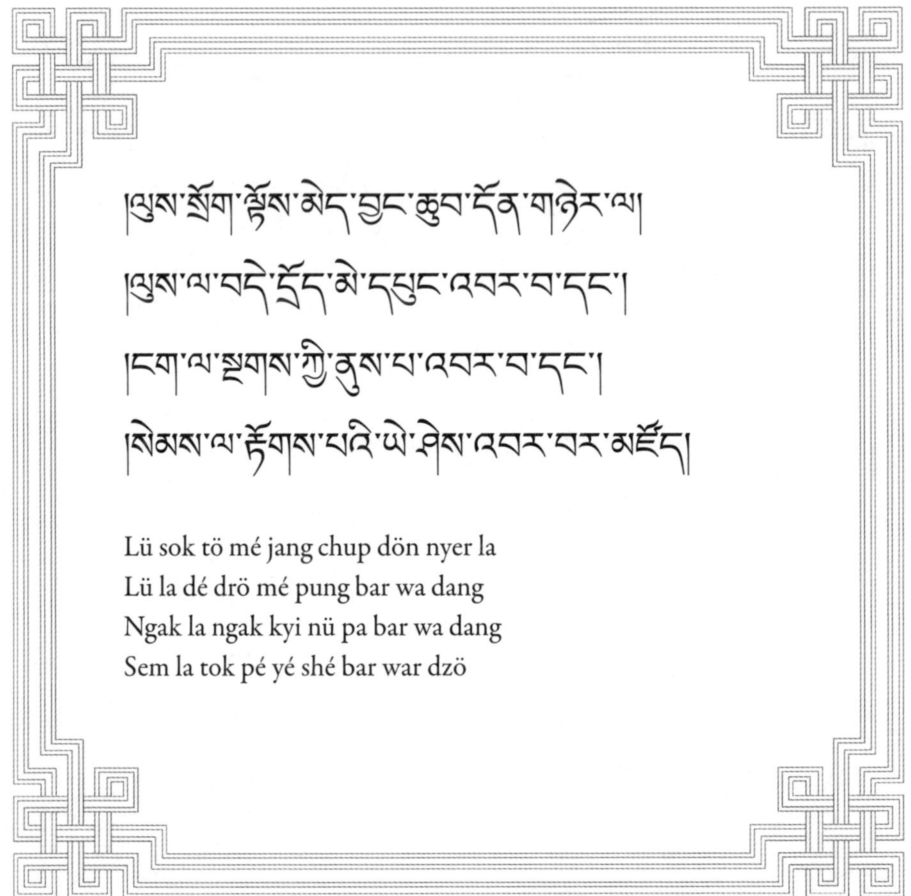

།ལུས་སྲོག་ལྟོས་མེད་བྱང་ཆུབ་དོན་གཉེར་ལ།
།ལུས་ལ་བདེ་དྲོད་མེ་དཔུང་འབར་བ་དང་།
།ངག་ལ་སྔགས་ཀྱི་ནུས་པ་འབར་བ་དང་།
།སེམས་ལ་རྟོགས་པའི་ཡེ་ཤེས་འབར་བར་མཛོད།

Lü sok tö mé jang chup dön nyer la
Lü la dé drö mé pung bar wa dang
Ngak la ngak kyi nü pa bar wa dang
Sem la tok pé yé shé bar war dzö

Without regard for body and life, I strive for enlightenment.
May the fireball of blissful heat blaze in my body!
May the potency of mantra blaze in my speech!
May the realization of primordial wisdom blaze in my mind!

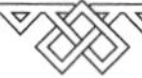

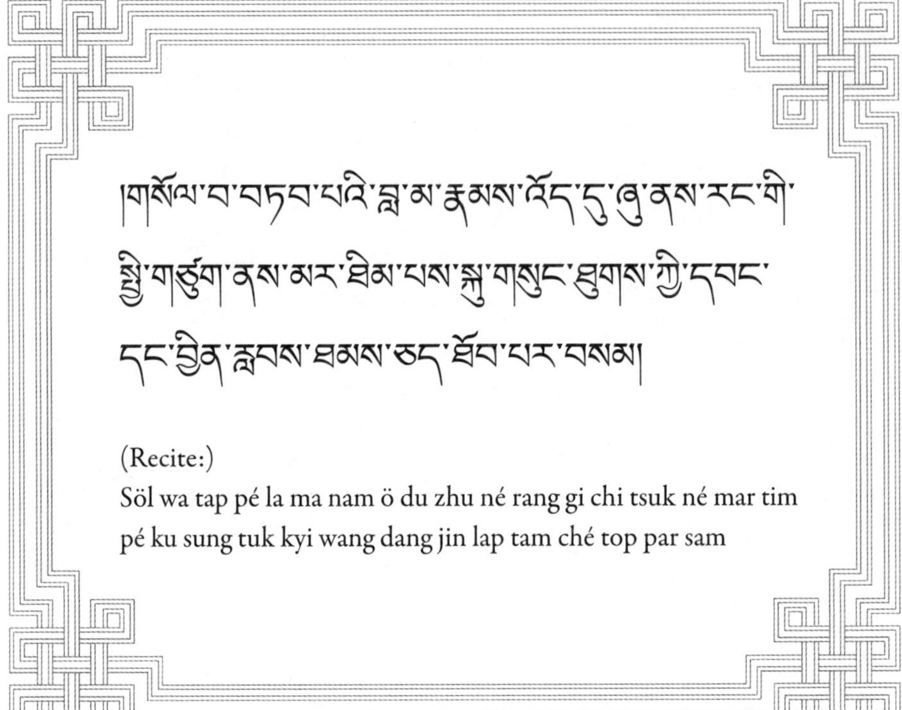

།གསོལ་བ་བཏབ་པའི་བླ་མ་རྣམས་འོད་དུ་ཞུ་ནས་རང་གི་
སྤྱི་གཙུག་ནས་མར་ཐིམ་པས་སྐུ་གསུང་ཐུགས་ཀྱི་དབང་
དང་བྱིན་རླབས་ཐམས་ཅད་ཐོབ་པར་བསམ།

(Recite:)
Söl wa tap pé la ma nam ö du zhu né rang gi chi tsuk né mar tim pé ku sung tuk kyi wang dang jin lap tam ché top par sam

(Recite:)
The lamas to whom I have prayed dissolve into light, which then dissolves down into the crown of my head. Through that, I obtain all the blessings and power of enlightened body, speech, and mind.

(Thus pray. Then, engage in *lung* practice. For the details of practice, look to your own texts. Visualize the lama dissolving into your crown, empowering your body, speech, and mind. If time permits, visualize the channels and perform the nine-round breathing practice.)

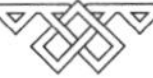

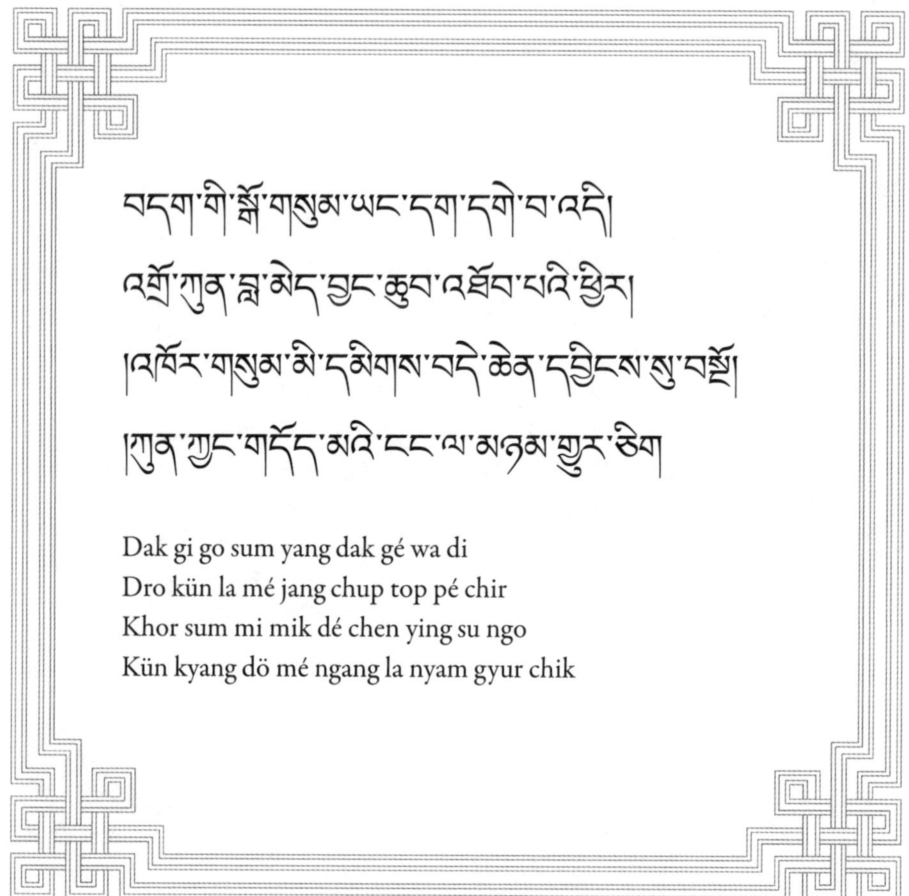

བདག་གི་སྒོ་གསུམ་ཡང་དག་དགེ་བ་འདི།
འགྲོ་ཀུན་བླ་མེད་བྱང་ཆུབ་འཐོབ་པའི་ཕྱིར།
།འཁོར་གསུམ་མི་དམིགས་བདེ་ཆེན་དབྱིངས་སུ་བསྔོ།
།ཀུན་ཀྱང་གདོད་མའི་ངང་ལ་མཉམ་གྱུར་ཅིག

Dak gi go sum yang dak gé wa di
Dro kün la mé jang chup top pé chir
Khor sum mi mik dé chen ying su ngo
Kün kyang dö mé ngang la nyam gyur chik

Concluding Practice

Dedication and Aspiration

I dedicate all this perfect virtue of my three doors,
So that all sentient beings may obtain unsurpassable enlightenment.
I dedicate this within the nonreferential blissful space, which is free of the three spheres of subject, object, and action.
May all become equal with the primordial state!

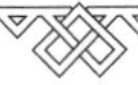

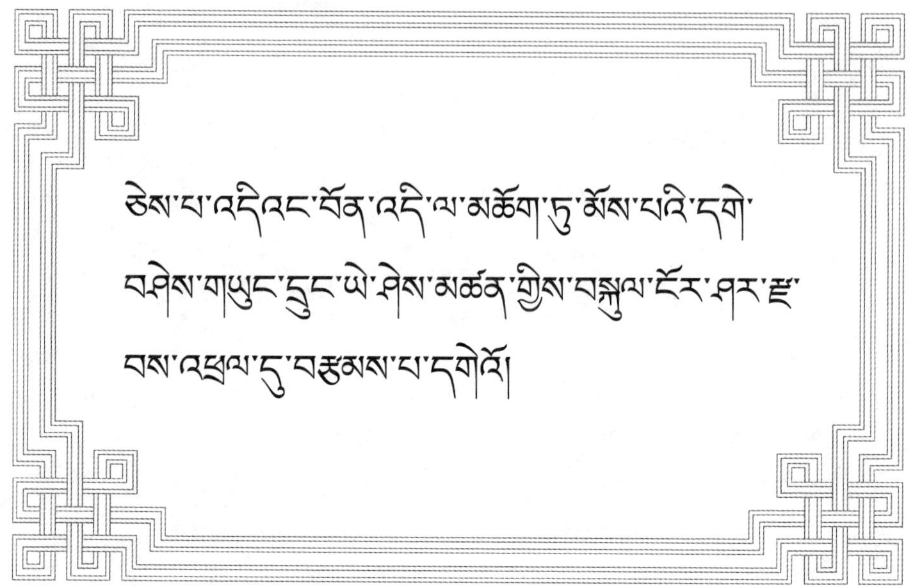
ཅེས་པ་འདིའང་བོན་འདི་ལ་མཆོག་ཏུ་མོས་པའི་དགེ་
བཤེས་གཡུང་དྲུང་ཡེ་ཤེས་མཚན་གྱིས་བསྐུལ་ངོར་ཤར་རྫ་
བས་འཕྲུལ་དུ་བརྩམས་པ་དགེའོ།

This was composed spontaneously by Shardza at the request of Geshe Yungdrung Yeshe who has supreme faith in Bön. Virtue!

Auspiciousness! Victory!

This text is from pages 101 to 104 of Shardza Tashi Gyaltsen's Dzogchen: The Self-Arising of the Three Enlightened Bodies, *Volume 11, in the modern typeset edition, or it may be found in Volume 282 of the Tengyur as described on page 112 of "A Handlist of the Bönpo Kangyur and Tengyur" by Kurt Keutzer and Kevin O'Neill in* Revue d'Etudes Tibétaines, *Volume 17: http://himalaya.socanth.cam.ac.uk/collections/journals/ret/pdf/ret_17.pdf. This translation from Tibetan into English was done by Kurt Keutzer and Geshe Chaphur Lhundup and enhanced by comments from Laura Shekerjian. The Tibetan text was entered and the translation formatted by Kevin O'Neill. We gratefully acknowledge the prior translations of Raven Cypress Wood and Alejandro Chaoul.*

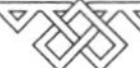

Bibliography

Tibetan Texts

Dru Gyalwa Yungdrung (Bru rgyal ba G.yung drung). *Magical Movements Stages that Clear Away the Obstacles* (*Gegs sel 'phrul 'khor rim*). In *Experiential Transmission of Zhang Zhung* (*Nyams rgyud rgyal ba'i phyag khrid bzhugs so*). 253–64. Edited by Dra rtsa Bstan 'dzin dar rgyas. Kathmandu: Triten Norbutse Bonpo Monastery, 2002.

Gyaltsen, Shardza Tashi (Rgyal mtshan Shar rdza bkra shis). *Magical Movements, Channels, and Winds of the Aural Transmission of Zhang Zhung* (*Snyan rgyud rtsa rlung 'phrul 'khor*, here referred to as the *Commentary*). In *Most Profound Great Sky Treasury* (*Byang zab nam mkha' mdzod chen*). 3: 321–46. Edited by Sonam N, Gyaltsen PLS, Gyatso K. New Thobgyal: Tibetan Bonpo Monastic Centre, 1974.

———. *Mass of Fire Primordial Wisdom: Bringing into Experience the Common Inner Heat* (*Thun mong gtum mo'i nyams len ye shes me dpung*, here referred to as *Mass of Fire*). In *Great Completeness Cycle of Instructions on the Three Self Dawning Dimensions* (*Rdzogs pa chen po sku gsum rang shar gyi khrid gdams skor*). 551–97. Delhi: TBMC, 1974.

———. *The Oral Main Points of Channels-and-Winds* (*Rtsa rlung gnad kyi zhal shes*, here referred to as *Main Points*). In *Most Profound Great Sky Treasury* (*Byang zab nam mkha' mdzod chen*). 3: 281–319. Edited by Sonam N, Gyaltsen PLS, Gyatso K. New Thobgyal: Tibetan Bonpo Monastic Centre, 1974.

Samlek, Milu (Rgyal gshen Mi lus bsam legs). *The Three Basic Mother Tantras with Commentaries* (*Ma rgyud sangs rgyas rgyud gsum rtsa 'grel*). Terma (*gter ma*) rediscovered by Guru Nontse (Guru rnon rtse) in the eleventh century CE. Reproduced from original manuscript belonging to Samling Monastery (bSam gling), in Dolpo, Nepal. Dolanji: Bonpo Monastic Centre, 1971.

Quintessential Instructions of the Oral Wisdom of Magical Movements (*'phrul 'khor zhal shes man ngag*, here referred to as *Quintessential Oral Instructions*). In *The Great Perfection Aural Transmission of Zhang Zhung* (*rdzogs pa chen po zhang zhung snyan rgyud*). In *History and Doctrines of Bonpo Nispanna Yoga.* Edited by Lokesh Chandra and Tenzin Namdak. Satapitaka Series. 73: 631–43. New Delhi: International Academy of Indian Culture, 1968.

Western Sources

Alter, Joseph S. "Modern Medical Yoga." *Asian Medicine: Tradition and Modernity* l, no. l (2005): 119–46.

Benson, Herbert, and Jeffrey Hopkins. "Body Temperature Changes During the Practice of gTum-mo Yoga." *Nature* 295 (21 January 1982): 234–36.

Chaoul, Alejandro. "Magical Movements (*'phrul 'khor*): Ancient Yogic Practices in the Bon Religion and Contemporary Medical Perspectives." PhD diss., Rice University, 2006.

———. *Tibetan Yoga for Health & Well-Being: The Science and Practice of Healing Your Body, Energy and Mind.* New York: Hay House, 2018.

———, et al. "Mind-Body Practices in Cancer Care," *Current Oncology Reports* 16, article no. 417 (2014). https://doi.org/10.1007/s11912-014-0417-x

———, et al. "Randomized Trial of Tibetan Yoga in Patients with Breast Cancer Undergoing Chemotherapy." *Cancer* 124, no. 1 (January 1, 2018): 36–45. https://pubmed.ncbi.nlm.nih.gov/28940301/

Cohen, Lorenzo, et al. "Psychological Adjustment and Sleep Quality in a Randomized Trial of the Effects of a Tibetan Yoga Intervention in Patients with Lymphoma." *Cancer* 100, no. 10 (May 15, 2004): 2253–60. https://pubmed.ncbi.nlm.nih.gov/15139072/

Engel, George L. "The Need for a New Medical Model: A Challenge for Biomedicine." *Science* 196, article no. 4286 (April 8, 1977): 129–36.

Karmay, Samten G. *The Little Luminous Boy.* Bangkok: Orchid Press, 1998.

Klein, Anne C. *Path to the Middle: Oral Madhyamika Philosophy in Tibet: The Spoken Scholarship of Kensur Yeshey Tupden.* Albany: State University of New York Press, 1994.

Martin, Dan. "The Emergence of Bon and the Tibetan Polemical Tradition." PhD diss., Indiana University, 1991.

Milbury, Kathrin, et al. "Couple-Based Tibetan Yoga Program for Lung Cancer Patients and Their Caregivers." *Psycho-Oncology* 1 (January 24, 2015): 117–20. https://pubmed.ncbi.nlm.nih.gov/24890852/

———, et al. "Tibetan Sound Meditation for Cognitive Dysfunction: Results of a Randomized Controlled Pilot Trial." *Psycho-Oncology* 10 (October 22, 2013): 2354–63. https://pubmed.ncbi.nlm.nih.gov/23657969/

Ong, Walter. *Orality and Literacy: The Technologizing of the Word.* London and New York: Methuen & Co., 1982.

Snellgrove, David. *The Nine Ways of Bon: Excerpts from the gZi brjid.* Boulder, CO: Prajña Press, 1980; second edition published by Orchid Press, 2009.

Wangyal, Tenzin Rinpoche. *Awakening the Sacred Body.* New York: Hay House, 2011.

———. *Tibetan Yogas of Body, Speech, and Mind.* Ithaca, NY: Snow Lion Publications, 2011.

White, David Gordon. *The Alchemical Body: Siddha Traditions in Medieval India.* Chicago, IL: University of Chicago Press, 1996.

About the Author

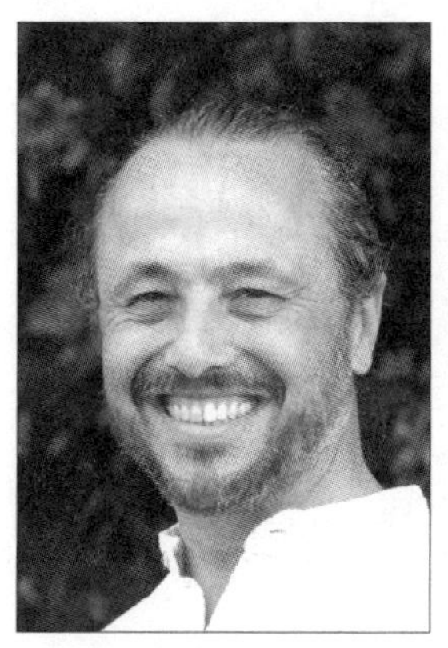

Dr. Alejandro Chaoul is a senior teacher at The 3 Doors, an international organization founded by Tenzin Wangyal Rinpoche with the goal of transforming lives through meditation. He has studied Tibetan yoga for thirty years with the Bön tradition's greatest masters, including the late H. H. Lungtok Tenpai Nyima, Yongdzin Tenzin Namdak, and Tenzin Wangyal Rinpoche, having trained in Triten Norbutse Monastery in Nepal and Menri Monastery in India. He completed the seven-year training at Ligmincha International and received his PhD in Tibetan Religions from Rice University. Since 1995, he has been leading meditation and Tibetan Yoga retreats throughout the United States, Latin America, and Europe under the auspices of Ligmincha International. Dr. Chaoul is the founding director of the Mind Body Spirit Institute at The Jung Center of Houston. He is the author of *Chöd Practice in the Bön Tradition* and *Tibetan Yoga for Health & Well-Being*.

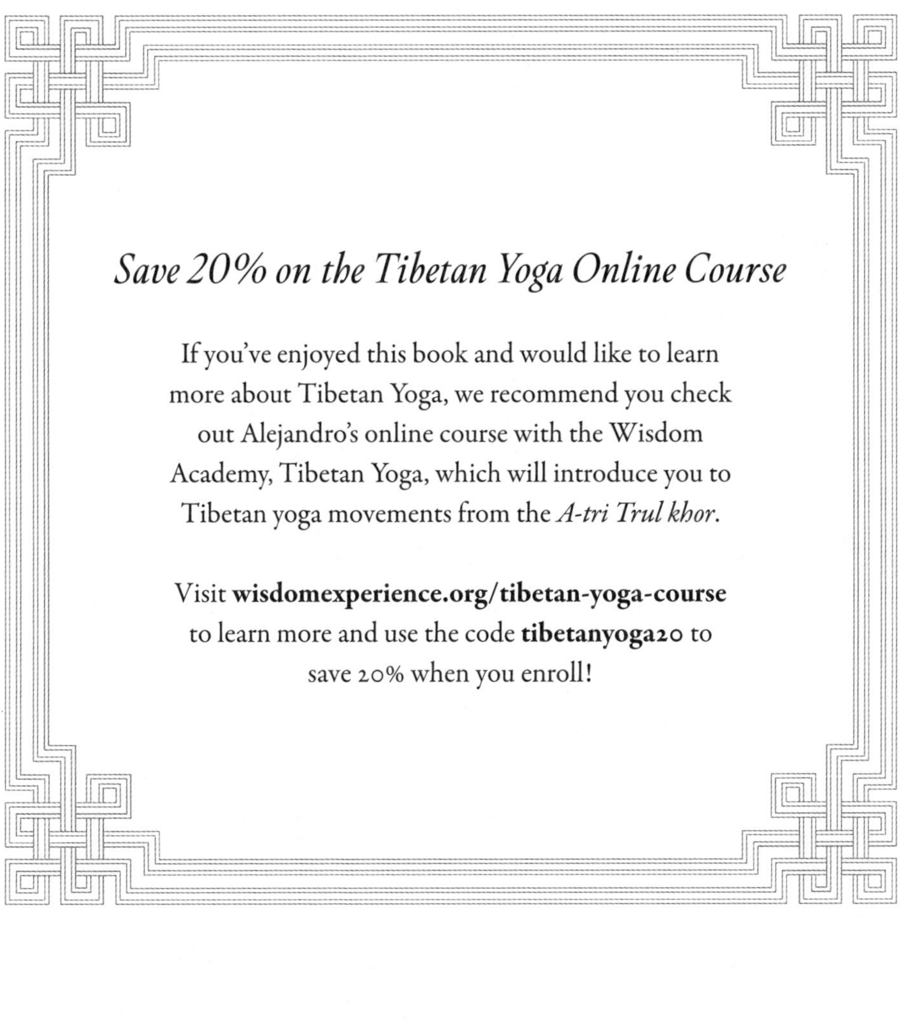

What to Read Next from Wisdom Publications

Mindfulness Yoga
The Awakened Union of Breath, Body, and Mind
Frank Jude Boccio

Editor's Choice—*Yoga Journal*

Veggiyana
The Dharma of Cooking: With 108 Deliciously Easy Vegetarian Recipes
Sandra Garson

"*Veggiyana* is more than just a cookbook—it's a feast in itself. It is a book to be treasured, living as it will in my kitchen and in my heart."—Toni Bernhard, author of *How to Be Sick: A Buddhist-Inspired Guide for the Chronically Ill and Their Caregivers*

Sit with Less Pain
Gentle Yoga for Meditators and Everyone Else
Jean Erlbaum

"Learn to sit in contemplative practice longer and translate simple yoga movements into creating ease in daily, routine tasks like sitting at a desk. Jean Erlbaum's well-informed book is straightforward and clear, with just enough detail for nonexperts."—*Yoga Journal*

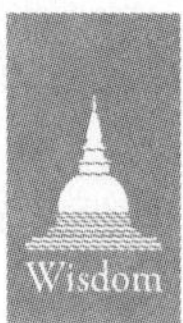

About Wisdom Publications

Wisdom Publications is the leading publisher of classic and contemporary Buddhist books and practical works on mindfulness. To learn more about us or to explore our other books, please visit our website at wisdomexperience.org or contact us at the address below.

Wisdom Publications
199 Elm Street
Somerville, MA 02144 USA

We are a 501(c)(3) organization, and donations in support of our mission are tax deductible.

Wisdom Publications is affiliated with the Foundation for the Preservation of the Mahayana Tradition (FPMT).